Professional Values in Nursing

Professor Lesley Baillie, PhD, MSc, BA (Hons), RN, RNT,
Florence Nightingale Foundation Chair of Clinical Nursing Practice,
Faculty of Health and Social Care, London South Bank University,
and University College London Hospitals

Dr Sharon Black, PhD, MA, PGCert, BSc (Hons), DipN, RN,
Programme Lead Nursing and Care Specialities,
Oxford Brookes University

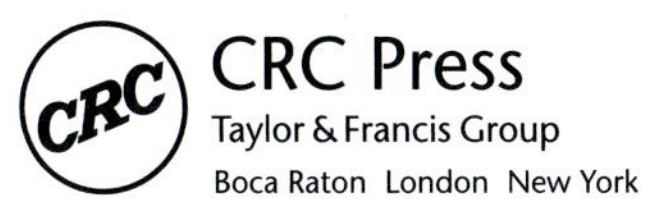

CRC Press
Taylor & Francis Group
Boca Raton London New York

CRC Press is an imprint of the
Taylor & Francis Group, an **informa** business

CRC Press
Taylor & Francis Group
6000 Broken Sound Parkway NW, Suite 300
Boca Raton, FL 33487-2742

Printed on acid-free paper
Version Date: 20140623

International Standard Book Number-13: 978-1-4441-8061-9 (Paperback)

Library of Congress Cataloging-in-Publication Data

Baillie, Lesley, author.
Professional values in nursing / Lesley Baillie, Sharon Black.
p. ; cm.
Includes bibliographical references and index.
ISBN 978-1-4441-8061-9 (paperback : alk. paper)
I. Black, Sharon, 1973- author. II. Title.
[DNLM: 1. Nurse's Role--Great Britain. 2. Ethics, Nursing--Great Britain. 3. Nursing--standards--Great Britain. WY 87]

RT85
174.2'9073--dc23 2014022610

Visit the Taylor & Francis Web site at
http://www.taylorandfrancis.com

and the CRC Press Web site at
http://www.crcpress.com

Contents

Contents

Contents

Contents

Foreword

Being a registered nurse is an honour and privilege, not only offering advice and guidance to the public seeking a healthy lifestyle but also intimately interacting with individuals and their families when at their most needy, when vulnerable and often afraid.

From the day of entry into pre-registration nurse education, students must start to understand and accept that as nursing professionals they will have to develop professional values. Indeed, it is a salutary day when the progressing student nurse recognizes that his or her whole life, both professional and in many aspects personal, must be lived according to a professional code beginning with registration. Not only will the nurse's practice and all decisions made, whether clinical or managerial, need to be professionally sound and ethical, wherever possible underpinned by a sound evidence base, but the nurse must also withstand the judgmental scrutiny of the public and professional peers.

Those in the public have their own perception of what constitutes professional nursing practice, and it is increasingly difficult in a complex world of health care to meet individual needs and the varying public demands, often informed by the Internet and modern media. Students enter training as members of that public, bringing with them personal values and probably preconceived values of the profession they are entering.

Educators and clinical practice colleagues have up to three years to instil in these newcomers to the profession the values that not only will underpin their own practice throughout their careers but will also make them valued members of a multidisciplinary team. What pre-registration education aims to produce are professionals who understand the unique contribution of registered nurses and are able to challenge if at any time they are concerned about the practice of others.

The understanding, recognition, application and enforcement of nursing professional values by registered nurses not only leads to excellence in practice and indeed protection of the public but also allows all registered nurses to be proud of the profession to which they belong.

Professor Judith Ellis, MBE
PhD, MSc, BSc (Hons), PGCE, RN (Child, Adult)

Preface

In 2010, the Nursing and Midwifery Council (NMC) published *Standards for Pre-registration Nursing Education*, which specified competencies that student nurses must achieve to become registered nurses. The NMC's competencies are grouped in four domains:

- Professional values.
- Communication and interpersonal skills.
- Nursing practice and decision-making.
- Leadership, management and team working.

This book focusses on the first domain and aims to instil in student nurses an understanding of professional values and how they underpin attitudes and behaviour. Professional values are also integral to the competencies in the other NMC domains as nurses' communication and approach to the people they care for and their families, the way that nurses approach their practice and clinical decision-making, and how nurses work in teams and manage and lead nursing care, are all influenced by their underpinning professional values.

The generic standard for the NMC's professional values domain is the following:

> *All nurses must act first and foremost to care for and safeguard the public. They must practise autonomously and be responsible and accountable for safe, compassionate, person-centred, evidence-based nursing that respects and maintains dignity and human rights. They must show professionalism and integrity and work within recognised professional, ethical and legal frameworks. They must work in partnership with other health and social care professionals and agencies, service users, their carers and families in all settings, including the community, ensuring that decisions about care are shared.*
>
> *(NMC 2010, p. 13)*

The competencies within the professional values domain specify aspects of this standard in more detail with generic competencies that are applicable to all fields of nursing (adult, child, learning disability and mental health), and competencies with specific application to each field. This book not only focusses on the professional values from a generic perspective but also includes practice scenarios focussing on adults, children, young people and families, who have varied mental and physical health care issues and disabilities and are accessing care in a range of healthcare settings. The text includes material relevant to all fields of practice and reflects the NMC's stance that there are a set of generic competencies that all nurses must demonstrate.

Preface

In Chapter 1, we explore values for professional nursing practice and encourage you to reflect on your own personal values and to analyse these in relation to professional body values, organisational values and wider healthcare values, in particular, the National Health Service (NHS) Constitution values. The chapter examines some core nursing values with application to professional nursing practice, and we examine how nurses can practise in a holistic, non-judgmental, caring and sensitive manner.

The focus of Chapter 2 is on the professional requirements for being a nurse, in particular, practising within the NMC's (2008) 'Code: Standards of Conduct, Performance and Ethics for Nurses and Midwives' and the requirements for continuing registration as a nurse. We examine key principles of professional practice, including consent, confidentiality, accountability and delegation and record-keeping in professional practice.

Chapter 3 considers the expectations of professional nurses from a wider perspective, including the media and public's images of nurses, what the public and patient groups expect from nurses providing care and the NHS expectations of a registered nurse. The chapter analyses quality and safety in nursing practice from public perspectives, and we conclude by discussing how nurses can uphold and promote a positive image of nursing.

In Chapter 4, we explore concepts of ethical practice in nursing and discuss some key ethical principles, theories and models of ethics and examine these in relation to decision-making and dealing with ethical dilemmas in practice. The chapter assists you to recognise and address ethical challenges relating to people's choices and decision-making about their care and introduces you to the concept of advocacy.

There is a vast array of legislation that has an impact on health care and nursing practice, so in Chapter 5, we focus on nursing practice within legal frameworks. We examine the application of legal principles that enable you to act within the law when providing nursing care. We discuss the legal capacity to make decisions about treatment and care, which is an essential consideration in all aspects of health care. The chapter also includes an exploration of concepts of duty of care and negligence.

Chapter 6 explores dignity, a concept that is central to human rights legislation and contemporary health policy and integral to professional and ethical nursing practice. We discuss the meaning of dignity, the vulnerability of health service users and how the promotion or loss of dignity affects the experience of care. The chapter includes an analysis of how dignity is influenced during care experiences by the care environment and the attitudes and interactions of caregivers and how nurses can promote dignity in practice for people across the lifespan and in different care settings.

The focus of Chapter 7 is on person-centred and holistic nursing care; these are important concepts within professional nursing practice which we explore from a range of perspectives in different care contexts. We examine how nurses can work with people in a way that values and respects them as individuals, taking account of their individual needs, preferences and culture, to deliver care that is person centred and holistic.

Chapter 8 follows from Chapter 7 by focussing on working in partnership with people to address their healthcare needs. We explore the nature and benefits of partnership working with people who access health care. The chapter analyses key aspects of partnership working, including relationships, shared decision-making and empowerment.

In Chapter 9, we explore the roles and responsibilities of other health and social care professionals and agencies and the need to work collaboratively to meet the needs of people who are accessing health care. The chapter highlights the importance of nurses understanding and respecting the roles of other health and social care professionals and recognising the need to refer people to other professionals if necessary.

Chapter 10 focusses on vulnerability and introduces you to principles of safeguarding. We explore the nature of vulnerability, with particular reference to people who are accessing health care. The chapter explains concepts of abuse, harm and neglect with reference to children and adults and the key principles in safeguarding children and adults, highlighting the nurse's duty to safeguard those who are vulnerable. The chapter highlights that policy and legislation in this area are frequently redeveloped and amended so that nurses must continually update their knowledge in this regard.

In Chapter 11, we focus on the need to challenge and report discrimination and poor standards of care and working practices. The chapter explores whistle-blowing in the light of legal, ethical and professional duties to report concerns. We examine the skills and courage that nurses require to communicate concerns, deal with confidentiality dilemmas and report colleagues.

Chapter 12 examines the professional requirement for nurses to engage with lifelong learning and deliver and promote care that is based on the best-available evidence. We consider how nurses can access, appraise and implement best evidence for practice. The chapter also explains how nurses can develop as professionals from the point of registration, including the role of preceptorship, clinical supervision and appraisal.

Preface

Our aim for this book is to support student nurses to develop a depth of understanding of professional values in nursing practice, from the start of the nursing course until the point of registration. The book also supports the transition from being novice students to registered nurses, with professional values embedded in nursing practice. Throughout the book, we refer you to other resources (books, journal papers, health policy documents, professional guidance and Internet sites) so that you can consider specific concepts in further depth. Each chapter starts with an introduction and learning outcomes. The chapters explore their topic, providing a strong evidence base, including theory and research, and references to key professional and policy documents. We include reflective and practice-based activities, as we aim that you apply the reading to your own practice and experience, which will help you understand professional values in nursing practice. Each chapter ends with a summary and the references used in the chapter, with recommendations for further reading and other resources to extend learning if available.

We hope that this book will make a valuable contribution to your learning and understanding of professional values in nursing. We wish you well in your nursing studies and your future careers.

Lesley Baillie and Sharon Black

References

Nursing and Midwifery Council. 2008. *The Code: Standards for Conduct, Performance and Ethics for Nurses and Midwives*. London: NMC.

Nursing and Midwifery Council. 2010. *Standards for Pre-registration Nursing Education*. London: NMC.

1 Values for professional nursing practice: an introduction

Introduction

Rassin (2008) asserted that:

> *Values lie at the core of the diverse world of human behaviour and are expressed in every human decision and action.*
>
> (p. 614)

Values are important in nursing and health care as they underpin all aspects of professional practice, including decision-making. This chapter explores values for professional nursing practice and encourages you to reflect on your own personal values and to analyse these in relation to professional body and wider healthcare values. We examine how values influence attitudes and underpin health care and professional nursing practice. We introduce some core values for nursing and explore how nurses can practise in a holistic, non-judgemental, caring and sensitive manner.

Learning outcomes

By the end of this chapter, you will be able to

- Analyse the nature of values and how values influence attitudes and behaviour;
- Discuss personal, professional and organisational values in relation to health care and professional nursing practice;
- Reflect on how nurses can practise in a holistic, non-judgemental, caring and sensitive manner.

The nature of values

There is an increasing emphasis on the importance of values in healthcare practice. We will start by exploring the meaning of *value* and some related concepts.

Activity

Consider:

- What is a 'value', and what is a 'belief'? How do they differ? How do emotions relate to beliefs and values?
- Look up definitions for *belief*, *value* and *emotion* in a dictionary and consider how the definitions you read compare with your own thoughts.

Dictionary definitions refer to a *belief* as having confidence that something is true. Beliefs can be influenced by many factors, including knowledge, experience, upbringing, culture, and religion. An *emotion* is usually defined as a feeling, for example, sadness, anger, joy, or fear. Our beliefs often affect our emotions and in turn our behaviour; see the practice scenario in Box 1.1 for an example that we explore further in relation to professional values.

Box 1.1

Practice scenario: how beliefs affect emotions and behaviour

Kelly and Dean's first son, Alfie, is nearly a year old. They tell their health visitor that they do not want to take Alfie for his MMR (mumps, measles, rubella) injection (*behaviour*) as they are frightened (*emotion*) that the injection might cause autism. When asked for their reasons, they say that they have read that MMR injections are a cause of autism, and also they know someone whose child developed autism after receiving the MMR (*belief*).

Dictionary definitions of *value* often refer to principles or beliefs that influence behaviour. Similarly, the Ethics Resource Center (2009) defines values as 'Core beliefs that guide and motivate attitudes and actions'. This definition implies a close connection between beliefs and values and that values influence our attitudes and behaviour. Rokeach (1973) has studied the nature of human values in depth and proposed the following definition:

> *An enduring belief that a specific mode of conduct or end-state of existence is personally or socially preferable to an opposite or converse mode of conduct or end-state of existence.*
>
> *(p. 5)*

Rokeach (1973) acknowledged that although values tend to be stable, they can change or develop. He argued that values have cognitive, affective and behavioural components: what a person thinks is desirable; what a person feels is desirable; and the action that results from these thoughts and feelings. Writing from a nursing ethics perspective, Rassin (2008) suggested that values represent 'basic convictions of what is right, good or desirable, and motivate both social and professional behaviour' and that values therefore provide 'standards for living' (p. 614).

Figure 1.1 portrays how values influence attitudes and how they together influence professional behaviour, including prioritisation of care and quality of care provided. We should also recognise that care quality is influenced not only by individual behaviour but by organisational culture, which we explore in more detail further in this chapter.

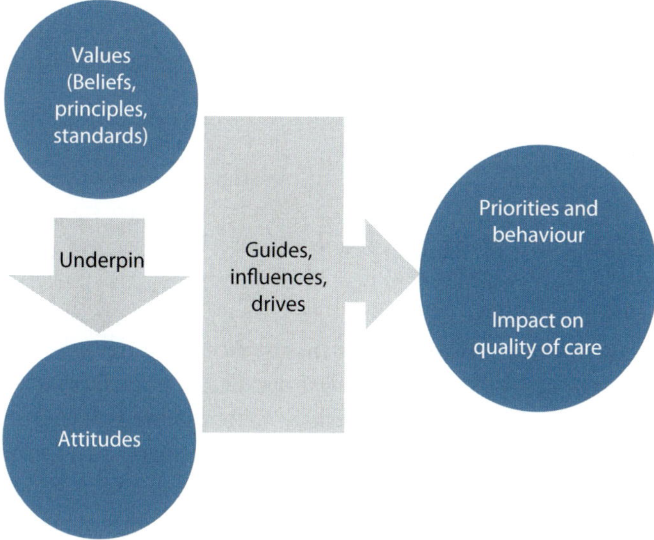

Figure 1.1 Values, attitudes and behaviour in professional practice.

If we understand the beliefs and values of people who we care for, we can better understand their behaviour and respect them as individuals. To return to Box 1.1, the National Health Service (NHS) recommendation, based on the evidence available, is that children should have the MMR vaccine, and there is no evidence for a link between MMR vaccine and autism, although this claim was widely publicised in the media (see http://www.nhs.uk/Conditions/vaccinations/Pages/mmr-questions-answers.aspx#autismrisk). The health visitor must adopt a non-judgemental and sensitive stance and recognise Kelly and Dean's fears and their desire to do the best for their child, which underpins their behaviour. The health visitor has a professional duty to ensure that Kelly and Dean have the most accurate information on which to base their decision, and this is best achieved through being respectful towards them and taking a partnership approach (see Chapter 8). Nurses must be sensitive to beliefs and values and respond respectfully.

Personal values

The Nursing and Midwifery Council's (NMC's) Essential Skills Cluster for 'care, compassion and communication' recommends that the newly qualified graduate nurse has 'insight into own values and how these may impact on interactions with others' (NMC 2010, p. 109).

Activity

- Reflect on your personal values and list four or five that are important to you in your everyday life.
- How could these values affect your attitudes and behaviour towards people you care for as a nurse?

As an example, in a study based in Sweden, Naden and Eriksson (2004) found that nurses whose behaviour promoted dignity had a strong moral attitude that was underpinned by values such as respect, honesty and responsibility; such nurses had a 'genuine interest and desire to help patients' (p. 90). Box 1.2 provides a practice scenario and asks you to consider the values underpinning the nurse's behaviour in practice. The nurse's values could include courage, compassion, concern, determination, empathy, fairness, kindness and respect. You may identify other values that underpinned her practice and influenced her stance in this situation. It is important to recognise the plight of other patients waiting on trolleys for beds on wards. However, the nurse recognised that for her patient, a temporary move to the discharge lounge would have been particularly distressing.

Box 1.2

Practice scenario: values underpinning nursing practice

A man who had moderately severe dementia had a lengthy stay in an acute hospital ward while he waited for a care home placement. On the morning of his discharge to the care home, a staff nurse took a telephone call from a bed manager who told her that the man must be moved to the discharge lounge to await his transport to the care home. The staff nurse argued that the man had a difficult and confusing day ahead of him and that it was unfair to move him to an unfamiliar environment with staff who he did not know and with whom he had no relationship. The manager applied a great deal of pressure, saying that there were patients lying on trolleys in the emergency department, but the nurse stood her ground. Eventually, the manager agreed that the man should wait for his transport on the ward and that she would find another patient who would find a temporary move less distressing.

Question:

What values might have influenced the staff nurse's behaviour?

In a less positive example of how values relate to attitudes and behaviour, student nurses described how older patients with dementia were 'treated as second class citizens' in acute hospital wards (Baillie et al. 2012, p. 35). Negative attitudes were particularly likely where the patients did not 'fit' in the acute ward; for example, one student said:

> *They always see them as a nuisance and "why are they here, there's nothing medically wrong with them"? ... The attitude of staff is often that they're just in the way, there's more critically ill patients. So they get ignored and left to the end.*
>
> (Baillie et al. 2012, p. 35)

We should question why hospital staff might consider patients with dementia, who may be vulnerable, confused and afraid, as less deserving of care than other, more acutely ill patients and what might have influenced the development of these attitudes and their underlying values. The next section explores the influences on personal values.

Influences on personal values

Increasingly, there are calls for assessment of the personal values of people recruited to healthcare courses (National Commission on Dignity in Older People 2012; Francis Inquiry 2013), the idea being to select people with the 'right' values to work in health care. According to Rokeach (1973), values are learned criteria, but where do we learn values from?

Activity

Look back at the previous activity that asked you to identify your personal values. Now consider the following:

- Where did your values come from?
- What influenced their development?

Rokeach (1973) identified culture, society (including its institutions) and personality as key antecedents of human values. You might have identified other influences, such as your family and your upbringing, your friends, a religion/belief system, your culture, the media, your education, and your life experiences. As regards the previous example of negative attitudes towards older people with dementia, many writers question whether older people are valued in society and whether the prevailing attitudes of society have an impact on health care. For example, Chan and Chan (2009) asserted that ageism and stigmatisation of people with dementia is embedded in society and reflected in UK care systems. Your values in relation to older people, and specifically those with dementia, could be influenced by your family, your culture, or your life experiences. You might also consider the influence of the media.

Activity

Look at some recent newspapers and think about television programmes that you watch. Consider:

- What are the images portrayed of different groups of people in our society?
- Which images are positive and which are negative?

Pay particular attention to how people of different ages (children, teenagers, older people) and people with disabilities are referred to in the media.

Did you notice any differences between media images of young children and those of teenagers, who are sometimes demonised by the press? What did you notice about how older people are presented? McSherry and Coleman (2011) observed that:

> *Older people can often be left feeling useless and unwanted in a society that seems to value youthfulness and beauty over wisdom, experience, knowledge.* *(p. 111)*

A report from the Commission on Dignity in Care (2012) also noted:

> *Undignified care of older people does not happen in a vacuum; it is rooted in the discrimination and neglect evident towards older people in British society.* *(p. 8)*

Rassin (2008) identified that key factors influencing nurses' values include professional education, training and experience, although there are varied opinions regarding whether experience can change personal and professional values. You might consider the effect on students of exposure to negative attitudes in a practice setting, for example, the negative attitudes displayed towards people with dementia cited previously. Negative attitudes may be translated into poor practice; if you witness poor practice, you have a duty to raise your concerns (see Chapter 11, which focusses on how to do this).

Activity

Reflect on what you have learned from your nursing education and experience in practice so far. Has this affected your values in any way? Has any of your learning or experience

- Challenged your values?
- Changed your values?
- Confirmed your values?

During your nursing course, you will learn about the values of the NHS, professional body values, and the values of the organisation where you practise as a student nurse. NHS values are considered next.

NHS values

There has been increasing emphasis on values within the NHS. In 2009, the Department of Health first published an NHS Constitution, which sets out rights and responsibilities for patients and NHS staff. In the current version of the NHS Constitution (DH 2013), the Department of Health sets out the intention to renew the Constitution every 10 years, with public, patient and staff involvement. The NHS Constitution's core values are: respect and dignity, quality of care, compassion, improving lives, working together for patients, everyone counts.

Activity

- Why might it be beneficial to have core NHS values? What benefits could there be for patients and the public and for the NHS workforce?
- How do the NHS core values relate to your own personal values, which you explored previously?

The NHS Constitution applies to a huge number of workers and although some, such as registered nurses, allied health professionals and medical staff, have their own professional codes which set out values, there are many unregistered NHS staff who have a crucial impact on patient experience, for example, catering staff, porters, and receptionists. To have core NHS values that apply to everyone working in the NHS could therefore establish a common view about what is important in care. However, they will only influence attitudes and behaviour if all staff have a common understanding of the values and actually apply them in their practice. Unfortunately, despite setting out the NHS values, there have been reports detailing unsafe and uncompassionate care (Health Service Ombudsman 2011; Francis Inquiry 2013). The 2013 Francis report expressed concerns that not all staff have yet taken on board the values expressed in the NHS Constitution:

> *The NHS Constitution is intended to be a common source of values and principles by which the NHS works, but it has not as yet had the impact it should. It should become the common reference point for all staff. ... All staff should be required to commit to abiding by its values and principles.*
>
> (*Francis Inquiry 2013, Vol. 3, p. 1399*)

The 6Cs

In 2012, the Department of Health in England carried out a widespread consultation exercise on values for nurses, which was published in 'Compassion in Practice: Nursing, Midwifery and Care Staff: Our Vision and Strategy'. The vision is based around six values: care, compassion, competence, communication, courage and commitment. The vision aims to embed these values (the 6Cs) in all nursing, midwifery and caregiving settings throughout the NHS and social care to improve care for patients. Box 1.3 presents brief definitions of these values, which were developed during the consultation. We next explore these values from some other perspectives.

Box 1.3

6Cs of caring*

Care

Care is our core business and that of our organisations, and the care we deliver helps the individual person and improves the health of the whole community. Caring defines us and our work. People receiving care expect it to be right for them, consistently, throughout every stage of their life.

Compassion

Compassion is how care is given through relationships based on empathy, respect and dignity—it can also be described as intelligent kindness, and is central to how people perceive their care.

Competence

Competence means all those in caring roles must have the ability to understand an individual's health and social needs and the expertise, clinical and technical knowledge to deliver effective care and treatments based on research and evidence.

Communication

Communication is central to successful caring relationships and to effective team working. Listening is as important as what we say and do and essential for 'no decision about me without me'. Communication is the key to a good workplace with benefits for those in our care and staff alike.

Courage

Courage enables us to do the right thing for the people we care for, to speak up when we have concerns and to have the personal strength and vision to innovate and to embrace new ways of working.

Continued

Box 1.3 (*Continued*)

6Cs of caring*

Commitment

A commitment to our patients and populations is a cornerstone of what we do. We need to build on our commitment to improve the care and experience of our patients, to take action to make this vision and strategy a reality for all and meet the health, care and support challenges ahead.

* From Department of Health. 2012. *Compassion in Practice: Nursing, Midwifery and Care Staff: Our Vision and Strategy*. Gateway reference 18479. London: DH, p. 13.

Care and compassion are also identified as being fundamental virtues necessary in nursing (see Chapter 4, Table 4.1).

All these values are important for people to have positive experiences of their nursing care. The need for **compassion** has been increasingly emphasised in the light of negative reports of healthcare experiences, many of which illustrated lack of compassion. Compassion entails the recognition of another's suffering (or need) and acting to relieve or address it. Goetz et al. (2010) defined compassion as

> *the feeling that arises in witnessing another's suffering and that motivates a subsequent desire to help.*
>
> *(p. 351)*

Sister Simone Roach (2002) was a Canadian nurse who studied caring in health care and she proposed 6Cs of caring (compassion, competence, commitment, conscience, confidence, comportment).

Roach (2002) argued that compassion is needed more than ever to humanise the ever-increasing cold and impersonal technology used within health care. Hudacek (2008) found that compassion required nurses to be present for patients both emotionally and physically and to focus on alleviating suffering and pain through empathic concern. In a study of compassion within the relationship between nurses and older people with a chronic disease, van der Cingel (2011) revealed seven dimensions of compassion: attentiveness, listening, confronting, involvement, helping, presence and understanding. This research highlighted that compassion is complex and multi-factorial.

Communication is essential for portraying compassion and building relationships. As regards **competence**, the NMC (2008) specified that nurses must provide a high standard of practice, displaying up-to-date knowledge and skills for practice to be safe and effective. Highlighting the importance of competent care, Roach (2002) stated that

> *while competence without compassion can be brutal and inhumane, compassion without competence may be no more than a meaningless, if not harmful, intrusion into the life of a person or persons needing help.*
>
> *(p. 54)*

Courage can be considered a value, but ethicists define courage as a virtue. Plato, the classical Greek philosopher (ca. 427–347 BCE) recognised four cardinal virtues of prudence, temperance, courage and justice; see Chapter 4 for an exploration of virtue ethics. Courage is important in nursing practice, for example, in relation to safeguarding people who are vulnerable (see Chapter 10) or raising concerns about standards of care (see Chapter 11). The NHS Constitution expects all NHS staff to raise concerns (Department of Health 2013); furthermore, it is a professional requirement for nurses to raise concerns about people who may be at risk (NMC 2008). Sellman (2011) argued that within today's healthcare system, where nurses must deliver safe and competent care within constrained resources, the need for nurses to be courageous, and remain firm to their values, is more important than ever.

Commitment as part of care requires that nurses will carry out necessary care in a consistent, reliable and timely way, regardless of barriers and constraints. Henderson et al. (2007) found that nurses needed to respond to patients' needs in a timely manner to be perceived as caring; patients were dissatisfied when nurses apparently forgot patients and their needs.

As a student you will spend 50 per cent of your course based in practice, in NHS trusts, the private sector or the voluntary sector. These organisations will have their own values, explicit or implicit, and you need to understand them. Organisational values are considered next.

Organisational values

Increasingly, NHS trusts and other healthcare organisations set out values that should guide behaviour in practice. The organisation will usually involve patients, the public and employees in identifying the values so that they are 'owned' by the organisation, rather than imposed. Box 1.4 provides an example.

Box 1.4

NHS trust values*

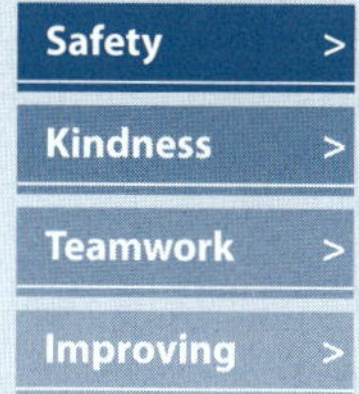

University College London Hospitals (UCLH) is a large NHS foundation trust in central London. The trust values of safety, kindness, teamwork and improving were launched in 2012. Around 1500 staff and patients were involved in the process of 'defining what embodies the very best of UCLH'. The trust applies the values in its recruitment and appraisal processes, and there are staff awards based on these values.

* From University College London Hospitals. 2012. *Official launch of trust values.* http://www.uclh.nhs.uk/News/Pages/6OfficiallaunchofTrustvalues28.aspx. Used with permission from UCLH.

While each ward, team or department should work within their organisation's values, they also are likely to have their own values, applied to their specific practice area. These local values may have been developed with the team and be explicit and displayed publicly. However, other teams may have implicit values, which underpin the ward/team culture and influence the social norms and accepted practices within the area. The ward or team culture in turn may have a positive or negative effect on the behaviour of individuals. For example, some wards have a culture of respect for patients (Baillie 2009). Leadership is highly influential in setting the culture.

In a study of student nurses' experiences of caring for older people with dementia in acute hospitals, some students found that spending time with patients was not necessarily acceptable within an organisational culture that valued speed above all else (Baillie et al. 2012). The students described that the priority was to move patients through the system quickly, so older people with dementia were repeatedly 'bumped from one ward to the next, to the next' (p. 34). Providing additional time for patients with dementia was often lacking as the focus was on treating the patient's physical condition: 'It's very treat the physical, very very treat the physical' (p. 35). However, the students recognised that: 'It was the emotional care that needs the attention' (p. 35).

Activity

- Find out about organisational values in the organisation where you are having practice experience:
  - Look firstly at the organisation's website: Are there any stated values or a vision statement?
  - When you are next on site, look for where the organisation's values are displayed: Can patients/residents/service users and families see them? Can staff see them?
- How do these organisational values relate to your own personal values and to the NHS Constitution values and the Department of Health's 6Cs? How do they differ and how do they inter-relate?
- When you are next on a practice placement, reflect on the local values of the ward/unit/team:
  - Are they explicit and displayed? If so, does the team's practice reflect these values?
  - Are there unstated values that underpin practice? If so, do these have a positive or negative influence on care delivery?

Professional body values

The NMC is the regulatory body for all UK nurses. As a nursing student, you must work within the NMC's (2008) *Code: Standards of Conduct, Performance and Ethics for Nurses and Midwives*, which is described as 'a shared set of values' and is applicable to all aspects of professional nursing practice. The Code is due for review in 2014, so ensure that you are familiar with the most current version, but the core values will remain stable. From looking at the Code, you will see that the focus is on behaviours, requiring that nurses treat people kindly and considerately, respect their dignity, respond to concerns and preferences, gain consent and involve people in decisions about their care. You will look in detail at the NMC Code in Chapter 2, and Chapter 6 focusses on promoting dignity in care. All registered nurses and midwives must behave according to the NMC Code, and as a student nurse, your behaviour should also align to this professional code.

Activity

Access the NMC Code on the NMC website and review it from the perspective of it as a 'shared set of values'. Identify some core underpinning values of the Code and then compare these with your previous activities, exploring

- your personal values,
- NHS values,
- organisational values.

In practice, you work within a multidisciplinary team. Allied health professionals and medical staff are registered with other professional bodies and must work within their professional codes. The Francis report (Francis Inquiry 2013) raised that different professions having discipline-specific codes could lead to a 'separation of cultural identity between different groups' and that NHS staff must remember that they are part of one large team with one objective: the proper care and treatment of their patients (p. 1401). In practice, there are many shared values expressed in the different regulatory bodies' codes of practice or ethics; some of these are considered in Chapter 9. In 2012 the NMC and the General Medical Council (GMC) released a joint statement on values to 'remind registrants of their professional values'. The statement included that

> *health professionals need to demonstrate compassion and kindness, as well as knowledge and skills. They have a duty to put patients first at all times and to raise concerns as soon as they believe patients are at risk.*
>
> *(Webpage)*

You will see that there is commonality between the values expressed in NMC's Code and the values within this joint statement from the NMC/GMC.

Professional values

Figure 1.2 portrays that your professional nursing values will be influenced by your personal values, but you should also be embedding into your practice the NHS, professional body and organisational values, which you

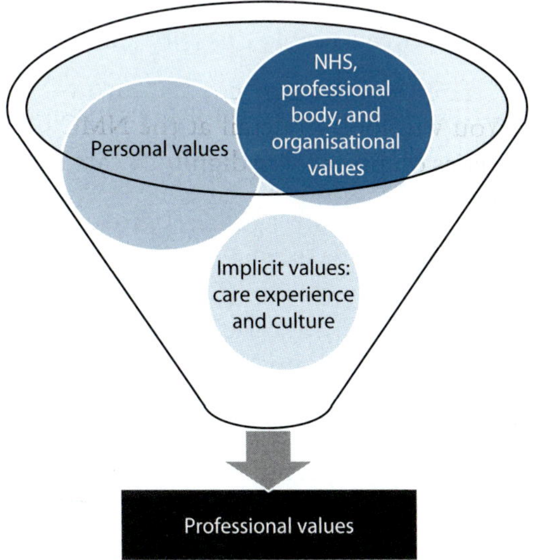

Figure 1.2 Development of professional values.

are learning as a student nurse. You should also be aware of the implicit values that you may encounter during health care experience, some of which may contrast with your own personal values and with the NHS and professional values discussed in this chapter. Badcott (2011) suggested that for individuals, there should be a minimal level of discord between their personal values in private life and the professional values for health care practice. He further suggested that when certain values are a condition of a particular profession, then these values must become integral to both personal and professional life.

Holistic, non-judgemental, caring and sensitive nursing practice

The NMC (2010) requires that graduate nurses are able to practise in

> *a holistic, non-judgemental, caring and sensitive manner that avoids assumptions, supports social inclusion; recognises and respects individual choice; and acknowledges diversity.*
>
> *(p. 13)*

This section explores these requirements.

To deliver holistic care, nurses need to consider the whole person and their physical, psychological, sociological and spiritual dimensions (Byatt 2008). Approaching patient care holistically helps to show respect for each patient as a person and a valued human being; see Chapter 7 for more exploration of holistic care. It is important to recognise the diversity of those we care for, in order to provide holistic care. Narayanasamy and Narayanasamy (2012) differentiated between visible diversity such as 'race', gender and physical characteristics, and hidden diversity such as sexual orientation, class and religion, which may not be obvious on first appearances but can affect care delivery. The UK's Equality Act (2010) established 'protected characteristics' within the legislation, which cannot be used as a reason to treat people unfairly; these are age, disability, gender re-assignment, marriage and civil partnership, pregnancy and maternity, race, religion and belief, sex, and sexual orientation (Equality Act 2010). The Equality Act should influence how society behaves towards people with 'established characteristics' and reduce discrimination. As such, the Equality Act is an important piece of legislation in relation to health care and nursing practice and is considered in more detail in Chapter 5. Professional codes, including the NMC's (2008) Code, also expect non-discriminatory behaviour.

If healthcare staff make judgements, as a result of personal biases, about those they care for, they may fail to see each person as a unique human being, resulting in prejudice in care delivery. The word *prejudice* means 'to pre-judge', rather than approaching each person as an individual. Often, prejudice results from stereotyping, which is the assigning of attributes to somebody because they are a member of a particular group (Walker et al. 2012), such as a certain ethnic group or age group or from a particular geographical location. Similarly, sometimes 'labelling' occurs, which is a type of stereotyping, for example, categorising people by aspects such as their behaviour or their age (Sale and Neale 2014). Higgins et al. (2007) found that prejudiced beliefs about patients were transferred from one nurse to another during handover and that colleagues' attitudes towards patients were influenced through informal communication and the use of stereotypical labels.

Activity

Reflect on your practice experience: Have you heard any labels used to describe patients? How might applying labels affect the approach of staff to patients?

Unfortunately, there is evidence of discrimination in health care; discriminatory behaviour from healthcare workers diminishes the dignity of patients (Baillie and Matiti 2013). A UK commission to investigate dignified care for older people highlighted that older people continue to experience discrimination despite being the major group of health service users (Commission on Dignity in Care 2012). There are many other people whose dignity and equality within health care has been found to be at risk because of discrimination, for example, gypsies and travellers (Peters et al. 2009), asylum-seekers (Asgary and Seger 2011) and people who are homeless (O'Donnell et al. 2007; Martins 2008). Deal (2007) suggested that overt prejudice towards disabled people seems to be disappearing in the United Kingdom but that subtle forms continue, to the detriment of the vision of disabled people being 'respected and included as equal members of society' (p. 93).

An independent inquiry into access to health care for people with learning disabilities (Sir Jonathan Michael and the Independent Inquiry into Access to Healthcare for People with Learning Disabilities 2008) highlighted inequalities. In a series of reports, Mencap, a UK charity campaigning for equal rights for children and adults with a learning disability, reported that people with learning disabilities continue to encounter direct discrimination from NHS staff who fail to treat them with dignity and respect (Mencap 2004, 2007, 2012). Mencap (2012) highlighted the legal requirement to provide equality in health care, so nurses must give the same quality of care and treatment to all patients, including those with a learning disability. Mencap (2012) suggested that discrimination occurs because of the lack of value afforded to the life of a person with a learning disability, indicating that, despite the Equality Act of 2010, the NHS values and professional codes of practice, some healthcare workers do not recognise the human dignity of people with learning disabilities. The Mencap (2012) report revealed cases in which nurses failed to provide even basic care to people with learning disabilities, neglecting nutrition, hydration and pain relief. In one scenario, in which a man with a moderate learning disability died after very poor care, a relative said:

> *I felt the nurses on the ward did not respect a gravely ill patient with special needs and a grieving family. Instead of using respect, tact, care and understanding, I and the rest of Alan's family were faced with hostility, disrespect and no consideration for the distressing situation.*
>
> *(Mencap 2012, p. 3)*

Many people have health conditions that carry stigma, and they are at risk of discrimination in their day-to-day lives. Nurses are in a good position to counter the discrimination they face and ensure that people who are vulnerable feel accepted and are cared for with sensitivity and respect. Box 1.5 gives one such example and includes some reflective questions.

Box 1.5

Practice scenario: applying values in practice

Lucy, aged 15 years, has developed severe depression. Recently she took an overdose of paracetamol and attended the emergency department for blood tests and treatment. Now back at home, her mother is frightened about what Lucy will do next. She is also embarrassed that Lucy has depression and has told her school that they must not tell Lucy's school friends why she is away from school. Lucy has now been referred to the CAMHS (Child and Adolescent Mental Health Services) team, and her mother accompanied Lucy to her first appointment. The nurse quickly put them at ease. After they returned home, Lucy's mother rang her sister and said how relieved she felt and that the nurse's attitude made her feel comfortable and accepted instead of anxious and ashamed.

Questions

1. Reflect on the NHS Constitution's core values of respect and dignity, quality of care, compassion, improving lives, working together for patients, and everyone counts. How might a CAMHS team apply these values in practice?
2. Think of examples of how the CAMHS nurse might have approached Lucy and her mother in a way that was warm, sensitive and compassionate.

Chapter summary

This chapter introduced professional values for nursing practice, and we have considered the nature of values and the many influences on professional values. You have explored your own personal values as a basis for understanding your attitudes and behaviour in nursing practice. You should now be familiar with the NHS values, the NMC's values and the values of the organisation in which you gain your practice learning experiences. There is now strong recognition that the values of individuals, teams and organisations have an impact on the attitudes and behaviours of healthcare staff and the priorities of organisations. Future chapters apply the concepts explored here in more detail in specific contexts.

References

Asgary, R., Seger, N. 2011. Barriers to health care access among refugee asylum seekers. *Journal of Health Care for the Poor and Underserved* 22(2): 506–522.

Badcott, D. 2011. Professional values: Introduction to the theme. *Medicine, Health Care and Philosophy* 14: 185–186.

Baillie, L. 2009. Patient dignity in an acute hospital setting: A case study. *International Journal of Nursing Studies* 46: 22–36.

Baillie, L., Cox, J., Merritt, J. 2012. Caring for older people with dementia in hospital: Part one: Challenges. *Nursing Older People* 24(8): 33–37.

Baillie, L., Matiti, M. 2013. Dignity, equality and diversity: An exploration of how discriminatory behaviour of healthcare workers affects patient dignity. *Diversity and Equality in Health Care* 10(1): 5–12.

Byatt, K. 2008. Holistic care. In Mason-Whitehead, E., Mcintosh, A., Bryan, A., and Mason, T. (eds.), *Key Concepts in Nursing*. Los Angeles: Sage, 168–174.

Chan, P.A., Chan, T. 2009. The impact of discrimination against older people with dementia and its impact on student nurses' professional socialisation. *Nurse Education in Practice* 9: 221–227.

Commission on Dignity in Care. 2012. *Delivering Dignity: Securing Dignity in Care for Older People in Hospitals and Care Homes*. Available from: http://www.nhsconfed.org/Publications/Documents/Delivering_Dignity_final_report150612.pdf (accessed 30 September 2013).

Deal, M. 2007. Aversive disablism: Subtle prejudice toward disabled people. *Disability and Society* 22(1): 93–107.

Department of Health. 2012. *Compassion in Practice: Nursing, Midwifery and Care Staff: Our Vision and Strategy* Gateway reference 18479. London: Department of Health.

Department of Health. 2013. *The NHS Constitution for England*. Available from: https://www.gov.uk/government/publications/the-nhs-constitution-for-england (accessed 24 November 2013).

Equality Act. Available from: http://www.legislation.gov.uk/ukpga/2010/15/contents (accessed 1 October 2013).

Ethics Resource Center. 2009. *Definitions of Values*. Available from: http://www.ethics.org/resource/definitions-values (accessed 3 September 2013).

Francis Inquiry. 2013. *Report of the Mid Staffordshire NHS Foundation Trust Public Inquiry*. Available from: http://www.midstaffspublicinquiry.com/report (accessed 1 September 2013).

Goetz, J.L., Keltner, D., Simon-Thomas, E. 2010. Compassion: An evolutionary analysis and empirical review. *Psychological Bulletin* 136(3): 351–374.

Health Service Ombudsman. 2011. *Care and Compassion? Report of the Health Service Ombudsman on Ten Investigations into NHS Care of Older People*. Available from: http://www.ombudsman.org.uk/care-and-compassion/home (accessed 1 September 2013).

Henderson, A., van Eps, M.A., Pearson, K., et al. 2007. 'Caring for' behaviours that indicate to patients that nurses 'care about' them. *Journal of Advanced Nursing* 60(2):146–153.

Higgins, I., van der Riet, P., Slater, L., et al. 2007. The negative attitudes of nurses towards older patients in the acute hospital setting: A qualitative descriptive study. *Contemporary Nurse* 26(2): 225–237.

Hudacek, S. 2008. Dimensions of caring: A qualitative analysis of nurses' stories. *Journal of Nursing Education* 47(3): 124–129.

Martins, D.C. 2008. Experiences of homeless people in the health care delivery system: A descriptive phenomenological study. *Public Health Nursing* 25(5): 420–430.

McSherry, W., Coleman, H. 2011. Dignity and older people. In Matiti, M., and Baillie, L. (eds.), *Dignity in Healthcare: A Practical Approach for Nurses and Midwives*. London: Radcliffe, 109–125.

Mencap. 2004. *Treat Me Right! Better Healthcare for People with a Learning Disability*. London: Mencap.

Mencap. 2007. *Death by Indifference: Following up the Treat Me Right! Report*. London: Mencap.

Mencap. 2012. *Death by Indifference: 74 Deaths and Counting: A Progress Report 5 Years On*. London: Mencap.

Naden, D., Eriksson, K. 2004. Understanding the importance of values and moral attitudes in nursing care and preserving human dignity. *Nursing Science Quarterly* 17(1): 86–91.

Narayanasamy, A., Narayanasamy, G. 2012. Diversity in caring. In McSherry, W., McSherry, R., and Watson, R. (eds.), *Care in Nursing: Principles, Values and Skills*. Oxford: Oxford University Press, 61–77.

Nursing and Midwifery Council (NMC). 2008. *The Code: Standards of Conduct, Performance and Ethics for Nurses and Midwives.* London: NMC.

Nursing and Midwifery Council (NMC). 2010. *Standards for Pre-registration Nursing Education*. London: NMC.

Nursing and Midwifery Council (NMC) and the General Medical Council. 2012. *NMC and GMC Release Joint Statement on Professional Values* Available from: http://www.nmc-uk.org/media/Latest-news/NMC-and-GMC-release-joint-statement-on-professional-values/ (accessed 1 October 2013).

O'Donnell, C.A., Higgins, M., Chauhan, R., Mullen, K. 2007. 'They think we're OK and we know we're not'. A qualitative study of asylum seekers' access, knowledge and views to health care in the UK. *BMC Health Services Research* 7: 75.

Peters, J., Parry, G.D., van Cleemput, P., et al. 2009. Health and use of health services: A comparison between gypsies and travellers and other ethnic groups. *Ethnicity & Health* 14(4): 359–337.

Rassin, M. 2008. Nurses' professional and personal values. *Nursing Ethics* 15(5): 614–630.

Roach, M.S. 2002. *Caring, the Human Mode of Being: A Blueprint for the Health Professions*. 2nd rev. edn. Ottawa: Canadian Hospital Association Press.

Rokeach, M. 1973. *The Nature of Human Values*. New York: Free Press.

Sale, J., Neale, N.M. 2014. The nurse's approach and communication: Foundations for compassionate care. In: Baillie, L. (ed.), *Developing Practical Nursing Skills*. Abingdon, UK: Francis and Wright, 33–74.

Sellman, D. 2011. Professional values and nursing. *Medicine, Health Care and Philosophy* 14: 203–208.

Sir Jonathan Michael and the Independent Inquiry into Access to Healthcare for People with Learning Disabilities 2008. *Healthcare for All: Report of the Independent Inquiry into Access to Healthcare for People with Learning Disabilities*. New York: Crown.

University College London Hospitals. 2012. Official launch of trust values. June 28. http://www.uclh.nhs.uk/News/Pages/6OfficiallaunchofTrustvalues28.aspx (accessed 22 April 2014).

van der Cingel, M. 2011. Compassion in care: A qualitative study of older people with a chronic disease and nurses. *Nursing Ethics* 18(5): 672–685.

Walker, J., Payne, S., Smith, P., Jarrett, N., Ley T. 2012. *Psychology for Nurses and the Caring Professions*. 4th edn. Maidenhead, UK: Open University Press.

2

Being a professional nurse: practising to the Code

Introduction

This chapter concentrates on the requirements of being a professional nurse and practising as a nurse who is registered with the Nursing and Midwifery Council (NMC). The chapter explains the role of the NMC in regulating professional nursing practice in the United Kingdom and what registered nurses must do to maintain their professional registration. The NMC's *Code: Standards of Conduct, Performance and Ethics for Nurses and Midwives* (2008) is introduced; a revised code is due to be published in 2014, but the core principles of being a professional nurse will remain constant. This chapter explores key aspects of being a professional nurse, including consent, confidentiality, record-keeping in professional practice, accountability and delegation. Legal perspectives specific to these areas of professional practice are referred to as appropriate; Chapter 5 focusses on legislation in more detail.

Learning outcomes

By the end of this chapter, you will be able to

- Explain the role of the NMC in relation to being a registered nurse and a nursing student;
- Discuss the NMC's Code and apply it to your professional practice;
- Explore key professional concepts of consent, confidentiality, accountability, delegation, and record-keeping in professional practice;
- Reflect on your own accountability and responsibility, recognising your limitations as a student and future registered nurse.

The Nursing and Midwifery Council and professional regulation

The NMC was established under the Nursing and Midwifery Order (2001) and came into being in April 2002, replacing the United Kingdom Central Council for Nursing and Midwifery (UKCC). The UKCC was set up in 1983 with the primary functions of maintaining a register of nurses, midwives and health visitors in the United Kingdom and managing professional misconduct. The NMC is the regulator for the largest group of healthcare professionals in the world, providing regulation for nearly 700,000 registered nurses and midwives. The primary purpose of the NMC is to safeguard the health and well-being of the public, and this is achieved by providing nurses and midwives with rules, standards and guidance on their professional practice. Even as a student, the NMC, your colleagues in practice and the general public expect you to behave in a professional manner at all times. It is only through demonstrating this professional behaviour that the public can have trust in you as a professional and have trust in the care that they receive.

The NMC exists to

- Safeguard the health and well-being of the public;
- Set standards of education, training, conduct and performance so that nurses and midwives can deliver high-quality health care consistently throughout their careers;
- Ensure that nurses and midwives keep their skills and knowledge up to date and uphold professional standards;
- Have clear and transparent processes to investigate nurses and midwives who fall short of the required standards.

The NMC also investigates and takes action on complaints against nurses and midwives when their practice has been called into question through complaints received from colleagues, the public, people in their care and other authorities.

Activity

The NMC has produced a YouTube channel. Visit this channel (http://www.youtube.com/nmcvideos) and look at the short videos NMC produced concerning safeguarding.

The NMC also has a Facebook page (https://www.facebook.com/nmcuk), which you can join and can then receive updates and be involved in discussions.

The NMC publishes a number of consultations relating to your practice, and it is important that you respond to these so that your voice is heard. The NMC is committed to engaging with patients, the public, registrants, students, employers, educators, other organisations and decision-makers.

Registering and maintaining registration with the NMC

To work as a nurse in the United Kingdom, you will have to register with the NMC. As a pre-registration nursing student, you will be registered in a nursing course that has been approved by the NMC. This means that your university will have gone through a process of approval with the NMC, which judges whether the nursing course the university developed meets the standards expected by the NMC. At the end of your course, if you have successfully met all of the requirements of that course, the university will submit your details to the NMC, and you will be issued a personal identification number (PIN) which is your licence to practise in the United Kingdom.

The NMC register is divided into three parts:

- Nurses
- Midwives
- Specialist community public health nurses

The nursing part of the register is divided into four fields of practice:

- Adult nursing
- Mental health nursing
- Learning disabilities nursing
- Children's nursing

Maintaining your NMC registration

The NMC requirements for maintaining your registration, summarised next, were up to date at the time of press. However, as professional requirements are regularly reviewed and updated, you must check the NMC website to ensure that these remain the most current available.

Every 3 years, usually on the anniversary of completing your pre-registration nursing course (although this date may change if you take a break from practice), you must renew your registration, called *periodic renewal*. You must also pay an annual fee at the end of the first and second years of your renewal period (check the NMC website on an annual basis to make sure you pay the correct fee). The NMC will notify you when your periodic renewal or annual retention is due. You must renew your registration every 3 years, for which you submit a signed notification of practice (NoP) form along with your renewal of registration fee. You must declare that you have met the Prep (post-registration education and practice) requirements (discussed further in the chapter) and are of good health and good character. Compliance with the Prep requirements, the professional standards set by the NMC, is a legal necessity. You will not be able to practise legally as a nurse if your registration lapses, so make sure you inform the NMC of any changes to your name or address so that you receive documents relating to your registration.

The NMC (2011) guidance for Prep aims to help registrants provide a high standard of practice and care, keep up to date with new developments in practice, think and reflect, and demonstrate that they are keeping up to date and developing their practice. The Prep standard's aim is to

> *safeguard the health and wellbeing of the public by ensuring that anyone renewing their registration has undertaken a minimum amount of practice.*
> *(p. 5)*

The NMC requires that you comply with its Prep requirements to renew your registration. You must complete an NoP form, which should declare the following:

- **You have practised as a nurse for a minimum of 450 hours** during the 3-year period (or you must have registered an additional nursing or midwifery qualification within the last 3 years). Practice can include administrative, supervisory, teaching, research or managerial roles and providing direct patient care.
- **You have undertaken and recorded at least 35 hours of learning activity relevant to your practice** during the 3-year period prior to renewal of your registration.
- **Any police charge, caution or conviction**, giving a clear account of the detail to the NMC.

You must maintain a personal professional profile of your learning activity and how it has informed and influenced your practice. The NMC conducts audits of registrants' Prep activity, and you must comply with any request to take part in the audit. Your evidence will need to be provided using Prep Continuing Professional Development (CPD) summary forms supplied by the NMC; these might include evidence from appraisals or course attendance certificates, so keep these safely so that you can find them when needed.

Revalidation proposals

The NMC is planning to introduce revalidation for nurses and midwives by the end of 2015. Revalidation entails the expectation that nurses and midwives regularly demonstrate that they remain fit to practise. The NMC (2013) identified the benefits of revalidation for the public, nurses and employers as the following:

- The public: enhanced public protection, better understanding of what to expect from nurses and midwives and increased confidence that nurses and midwives are fit to do their work;
- Nurses and midwives: ownership of the revalidation process and increased accountability, ability to use evidence to demonstrate CPD and that they meet NMC standards;
- Employers: ongoing engagement and a deeper understanding of the requirements of professional regulation; clarity on issues concerning conduct and competence.

The introduction of revalidation, or similar processes, applies more widely than nursing; the Department of Health (DH) and the Professional Standards Authority have recommended that a continuing fitness-to-practise measurement such as revalidation is necessary for all healthcare professions (NMC 2013). The NMC's proposed model of revalidation includes third-party input, with the view that this will give greater assurance, and there is strong support from patients and the public about including patient feedback as a part of revalidation to enhance public protection.

The NMC's (2013) proposal, currently under consultation, is for all registered nurses and midwives to be revalidated every 3 years when they renew their registration. They will need to gather evidence continually for their revalidation based on criteria in the updated Code and standards. At revalidation, nurses and midwives will confirm that they remain fit to practise; have met the required practice hours and CPD; have reflected on the updated Code and standards and continue to follow them; and have sought and received third-party feedback (from patients, carers or peers) which has informed their reflection on their practice. In addition, a third party (manager or supervisor) must confirm that the nurse or midwife is following the NMC's Code and standards and is fit to practise.

Professional indemnity insurance

Following EU legislation in 2013, from 2014 it is a legal requirement for all nurses (and all other healthcare professionals) to hold professional indemnity insurance (see http://www.nmc-uk.org/Registration/Professional-indemnity-insurance/). This insurance must reflect your scope of practice and the risks associated with your role. The purpose of this is to enable a patient to recover compensation if the patient has suffered harm because of a nurse's negligent action. Indemnity insurance can be obtained as follows:

- If you work in the National Health Service (NHS), the NHS will have indemnity insurance that will cover you, but you should check the details of this insurance.
- If you are employed outside the NHS, you should have coverage through your employer, but you must check that this is in place and check the details of this coverage.
- As part of membership in a professional body or trade union (the Royal College of Nursing [RCN], for example), coverage might be provided.
- Coverage can be obtained from a commercial provider.

It is your responsibility to check the details of this coverage, and if as a registered nurse you became self-employed, you must make sure that you can show evidence of your own indemnity insurance. You will be required to provide the NMC with evidence of indemnity coverage at the following times:

- When you register as a nurse for the first time;
- When you renew your registration;
- When you are applying to return to the register after a period away from being registered;
- If you are carrying out voluntary work for which you are practising as a registered nurse (check whether the voluntary organisation provides coverage; if not, then you must obtain your own).

The Code

The Code: Standards of Conduct, Performance and Ethics for Nurses and Midwives (NMC 2008) was developed primarily to safeguard the public. All nurses and midwives are expected to practise according to this Code, which can be found on the NMC website. Essentially, the Code lays out the behaviours and expectations required of you as a nurse. Through this Code, you are required to put the care of people at the forefront of what you do, which means treating people with dignity and respect, providing high standards of care, and protecting people when they are vulnerable.

Based on the Code, the NMC (2011) also produced guidance on professional conduct for nursing and midwifery students, and this should guide you on your journey to becoming a registered nurse. The guidance sets out the personal and professional conduct expected of you as a student. However, it is important that you know about both of the documents as a student so that you can appreciate what will be expected of you as a registered nurse when you graduate. There are four core principles reflected in both the Code and the guidance for you as a student:

- Make the care of people your first concern, treating them as individuals and respecting their dignity.
- Work with others to protect and promote the health and well-being of those in your care, their families and carers, and the wider community.
- Provide a high standard of practice and care at all times.
- Be open and honest, act with integrity and uphold the reputation of your profession.

Activity

Access the Code via the NMC website (http://www.nmc-uk.org/Nurses-and-midwives/Standards-and-guidance1/The-code/The-code-in-full/). Read the code and familiarize yourself with its content.

Reflecting on the definitions of values and beliefs outlined in Chapter 1, consider:

- How your personal values and beliefs fit with the Code;
- Whether your personal values and beliefs have to be modified to fit your professional code.

Throughout this book, you will find reference to the NMC Code as it is central to everything you do as a nurse, as are the chapters relating to ethics and the law. Some key aspects of the Code, including confidentiality, consent, record-keeping, accountability and delegation, are discussed in the next sections.

Confidentiality

A duty of confidence arises when one person discloses information to another (e.g. patient to clinician) in circumstances for which it is reasonable to expect that the information will be held in confidence (DH 2003). In your practice, confidentiality is a legal obligation derived from statute law and case law, and it will also usually be included in your contract of employment as a nurse, with a specific link to disciplinary procedures if breached.

Respecting confidentiality relates to you as an individual and to all NHS organisations. In 1997, a review was commissioned by the chief medical officer of England because of growing concerns about the way in which patient information was being used in the NHS and a need to protect and promote principles of confidentiality in an age in which technology enabled the rapid and widespread sharing of patient information. Dame Fiona Caldicott carried out the review, and her findings, the 'Caldicott Principles', were published in 1997 (DH 1997) as 16 recommendations that NHS organisations were required to adhere to and 6 principles for handling confidential information. In September 2013, the DH produced revised Caldicott Principles (DH 2013) (see Table 2.1).

Table 2.1 Caldicott Principles

Principle	Guidance underpinning principle
1. Justify the purpose(s).	Every proposed use or transfer of personal confidential data within or from an organisation should be clearly defined, scrutinised and documented, with continuing uses regularly reviewed, by an appropriate guardian.
2. Do not use personal confidential data unless absolutely necessary.	Personal confidential data should not be included unless the data are essential for the specified purpose(s) of that flow. The need for patients to be identified should be considered at each stage of satisfying the purpose(s).
3. Use the minimum necessary personal confidential data.	Where use of personal confidential data is considered to be essential, the inclusion of each individual item of data should be considered and justified so that the minimum amount of personal confidential data is transferred or accessible as is necessary for a given function to be carried out.
4. Access to personal confidential data should be on a strict need-to-know basis.	Only those individuals who need access to personal confidential data should have access to it, and they should only have access to the data items that they need to see. This may mean introducing access controls or splitting data flows where one data flow is used for several purposes.
5. Everyone with access to personal confidential data should be aware of their responsibilities.	Action should be taken to ensure that those handling personal confidential data—both clinical and non-clinical staff—are made fully aware of their responsibilities and obligations to respect patient confidentiality.
6. Comply with the law.	Every use of personal confidential data must be lawful. Someone in each organisation handling personal confidential data should be responsible for ensuring that the organisation complies with legal requirements.
7. The duty to share information can be as important as the duty to protect patient confidentiality.	Health and social care professionals should have the confidence to share information in the best interests of their patients within the framework set out by these principles. They should be supported by the policies of their employers, regulators and professional bodies.

Source: Department of Health, *Information: To Share or Not to Share, Government Response to the Caldicott Review.* 2013. Available from: https://www.gov.uk/government/uploads/system/uploads/attachment_data/file/239273/9731–2901141-TSO-Caldicott-Government_Response_ACCESSIBLE.pdf (accessed 17 October 2013).

Information provided by those in your care is given in confidence and therefore should be treated as confidential as long as it includes information identifying that individual. People in your care should be able to trust that you will keep their information safe and confidential, sharing it only with those involved in their care as necessary. It is important to make sure that any sharing of information is legitimate. The DH (2013) stated:

> *For the purposes of direct care, relevant personal confidential data should be shared among the registered and regulated health and social care professionals who have a legitimate relationship with the individual.*
>
> *(p. 14)*

However, the legal duty of confidentiality is not absolute, and there are a number of exceptions that will be highlighted in the following material.

The Data Protection Act (1998) is an act that made provision for the regulation of the processing of information relating to individuals, including obtaining, holding, using or disclosing such information. According to this act, you must use the sensitive information about those in your care 'fairly and lawfully'. In terms of your practice, you must inform the people in your care of the circumstances under which their confidential information will be shared (Data Protection Act 1998) and that this sharing is necessary to ensure they receive appropriate and high-quality care. This may not be obvious to them, so it may be necessary to highlight the members of the health and social care team involved in their care. You should also tell them that their information might be shared for the purpose of clinical governance processes and audits and for the use of other healthcare bodies as necessary.

The DH (2003) developed a confidentiality model (see Figure 2.1) to outline the areas that must be met to comply with the requirements of confidentiality, which will be useful to you in your practice if you are faced with uncertainty:

a. **Protect**: look after the patient's information;

b. **Inform**: ensure that patients are aware of how their information is used;

c. **Provide choice**: allow patients to decide whether their information can be disclosed or used in particular ways;

d. **Improve**: always look for better ways to protect, inform, and provide choice.

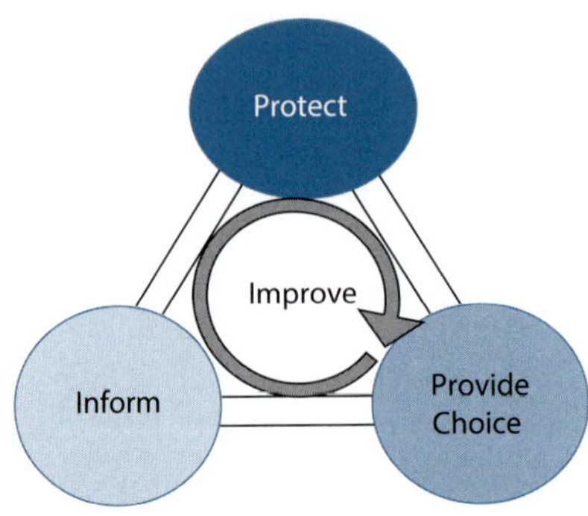

Figure 2.1 The confidentiality model. (From Department of Health, 2003. *Confidentiality: NHS Code of Practice*. London: Department of Health. Available from: https://www.gov.uk/government/uploads/system/uploads/attachment_data/file/200146/Confidentiality_-_NHS_Code_of_Practice.pdf. (accessed 17 October 2013).

When is it acceptable to breach confidentiality?

Confidentiality is protected in human rights law in Article 8 of the Human Rights Act (1998): the right to respect for private and family life, which states the following;

1. Everyone has the right to respect for their private and family life, their home and their correspondence.
2. There shall be no interference by a public authority with the exercise of this right **except** such as is in accordance with the law and is necessary in a democratic society in the interests of national security, public safety or the economic well-being of the country, for the prevention of disorder or crime, for the protection of health or morals, or for the protection of the rights and freedoms of others.

You will note that even in the Human Rights Act there are exceptions to protecting confidentiality. The Code (NMC 2008) does allow you to disclose information if you believe someone might be at risk of harm, in line with the law of the country in which you are practising. As a nurse, under common law, you are allowed to breach confidentiality in the public interest. This relates to the investigation and punishment of a crime, to prevent the abuse of others or to prevent harm. It is not possible to apply one rule in all cases; therefore, each case should be judged individually. In all cases, the public interest must outweigh the obligation to the individual concerned.

The term *public interest* describes the exceptional circumstances under which the right to confidentiality can be overruled to meet a broader social interest. If this breach relates to a person in your care, the decision to breach such confidence should not be taken alone. You should seek advice, and you must be able to justify the breach to the NMC or the courts, so it is important that you maintain clear records of the decisions you made and the process you went through. A leading case on disclosure in the public interest is that of *W* v. *Egdell* [1990] (see Box 2.1), from which the following guiding principle now exists in law:

> *Information may be disclosed in the public interest, provided that the risk is real rather than fanciful, and that it should involve the danger of physical harm to the public.*

Box 2.1

W v. *Egdell* [1990]

W was an inpatient in a secure hospital following convictions for killing five people and wounding others. He applied to a mental health tribunal to be discharged or transferred to a regional unit. An independent psychiatrist, Dr Egdell, was asked by W's legal advisors to provide a confidential expert opinion with the intention of proving that W was no longer a risk. They had hoped to submit this as evidence in W's application, but they withdrew the report from the tribunal because Dr Egdell was of the opinion that W was still a danger to the public and recommended that he stay in a secure unit. However, Dr Egdell felt that his report should be made known to the tribunal and therefore sent a copy to the secretary of state. W brought an action for a breach of confidence.

Although initially successful in the High Court, the Court of Appeal held that the breach was justified in the public interest on grounds of protection of the public from dangerous criminal acts.

Now, review the scenario in Box 2.2 and reflect on the questions in relation to the information in this section.

Box 2.2

Practice scenario: confidentiality

You are a nurse working in an accident and emergency environment. An 18-year-old male, Louis, attends with a stab wound to his arm. On assessing him, you find that he has a knife in his pocket which appears to have blood on it. Louis talks to you about a fight in which he was involved. He discusses how his family will be disappointed in him if he gets into trouble again (he has a previous conviction for assault) and is apologetic. He asks that you help him and that you promise not to tell anyone, which you do.

- On reflection, was this the right action to take? Should you have helped him and made that promise?
- What would be the consequences if you share this information with a colleague?
- What would the law say about such a breach of confidence? Under these circumstances, to whom do you owe the greatest duty of care?

If you apply the professional and legal requirements of confidentiality to the scenario in Box 2.2, there are two aspects to it. You are professionally bound to maintain confidentiality, and Louis can expect that his private life will be respected under human rights law; therefore you could be seen as doing wrong if you share this information. However, you have to make a moral decision under such circumstances. You will need to weigh whether the act of reporting this information outweighs the risks of you doing nothing (see Chapter 4 for further guidance on ethical decision-making). If you do nothing, you may be covering up a crime, and there is potential for further crime to be committed. You may feel sorry for Louis, but this is the first time you have met him and you know that he has committed a crime in the past. You need to be objective. You will be protected under the law of 'public interests' and under Article 8 of the Human Rights Act if you decide to breach confidence under these circumstances.

When considering the sharing of information for audit, teaching or research purposes, for example, once information is effectively anonymised it is no longer confidential. This nonetheless does necessitate the removal of all strong identifiers, such as name, address, postcode, NHS number or date of birth. The principles of sharing anonymised information are set in case law: *R* v. *Department of Health ex parte Source Informatics Ltd.* [2001] (see Box 2.3).

Box 2.3

R v. Department of Health ex parte Source Informatics Ltd. [2001]

Source Informatics, a company which sold information to drug companies, arranged for pharmacists and general practitioners (GPs) to pass information on to them. The information only included the GP's name and the prescribed drug. The DH issued guidance that anonymising information did not remove the duty of confidence and therefore asserted that this practice breached confidentiality, so Source Informatics sought a ruling against this decision.

The Court of Appeal decided that disclosing minimal anonymised information cannot amount to a breach of confidence because the patients' names and identifiers were removed.

Consent

Valid consent must be obtained from people in your care before any physical examination, treatment or provision of personal care; this consent reflects the right of people to determine what happens to their body (DH 2009). If this process is ignored, you may be liable to legal action and your employer may also be liable for your actions (DH 2009). The general principles of consent are set out in case law (common law). This has established that touching a person in your care without consent may result in a civil or criminal action for battery, or if you fail to obtain valid consent and the person in your care suffers harm, the person may bring an action of negligence (see Chapter 5) against you (DH 2009).

The DH produced a guide to consent for examination or treatment to direct English law (DH 2009). For that consent to be valid, it must be

> *given voluntarily by an appropriately informed person who has the capacity to consent to the intervention in question (this will be the patient or someone with parental responsibility for a patient under the age of 18, someone authorised to do so under a Lasting Power of Attorney (LPA) or someone who has the authority to make treatment decisions as a court appointed deputy).*
>
> *(p. 9)*

The consent must also be obtained without putting 'pressure' or 'undue influence' on that person so they can freely choose to accept or refuse that treatment or care (DH 2009). Any 'coercion' by a practitioner will invalidate the consent, as will the misrepresentation of the procedure; the person in your care must understand what the procedure or care involves and why that procedure or care is necessary for the consent to be valid (DH 2009). Whilst informing a person about the procedure or care facilitates valid consent and should prevent a claim of 'battery', there may still be cause for an action in negligence if that person then suffers harm (DH 2009).

In your everyday practice, you will see consent given to you in a number of ways. Consent may be **expressed** (involves the patient clearly expressing their wishes verbally or in writing); **implicit/implied** (inferred by the conduct of the person in your care; for example, they offer you their arm to have their blood pressure taken); **general** (covers possible 'blanket' agreements for treatment); or **specific** (consent should be related to a specific procedure) (Buka 2008).

Activity

Thinking about the care that you have witnessed and delivered, reflect on instances when you feel that consent was not obtained without some kind of influence from either a practitioner or a family member. For example, a practitioner, relative or carer might have said, "Take your medication or you will never get better". Also, think about whether consent is always gained before providing care and what type of consent this is.

Written consent only proves that the person receiving the treatment or procedure gave consent. It is still necessary to ensure the voluntary nature of the process of consent, that appropriate information was given, and that the person had the capacity to consent (DH 2009). The completion of a written consent form is only a legal requirement under the Mental Health Act of 1983 and the Human Fertilisation and Embryology Act of 2008; however, it is seen as best practice when a procedure such as surgery is performed (DH 2009). This best practice also relates to gaining written consent for participation in research (DH 2009).

When gaining consent from a person in your care, you should not assume that they have the knowledge to understand what you are saying. It is important that you give them enough time to consider the information and give them opportunity to ask questions. If, after considering the information, they decline the treatment or procedure, then you must respect their wishes to do so. If you obtain consent by failing to give an appropriate amount of information or by deceiving a person in your care, this could result in an allegation of battery (or civil assault).

Capacity and autonomy are central to the concept of consent. Capacity to consent is enshrined in the Mental Capacity Act of 2005, which is discussed in greater detail in Chapter 5. The capacity of people in your care to make informed choices may or may not be compromised by the nature of their illness or treatment, but they should all be afforded the opportunity to make informed choices about their care and treatment if possible. This applies not only to medical treatment but also to the day-to-day procedures and care that you give as a nurse.

You are responsible for checking that the people in your care have actually consented to procedures even if you are not accountable for taking that consent (i.e. consent for surgery). As a nurse you are in a good position to know what information a person in your care will require for the consent to be legal and valid. If you are concerned about a person's understanding of a procedure, you should communicate this to the team. The NMC (2013) outlined three over-riding professional responsibilities for nurses in relation to consent:

- To make the care of people their first concern and ensure they gain consent before they begin any treatment or care;
- Ensure that the process of establishing consent is rigorous and transparent and demonstrates a clear level of professional accountability;
- Accurately record all discussions and decisions relating to obtaining consent.

Now, read the scenario in Box 2.4 and consider the questions.

Box 2.4

Practice scenario: consent

You are caring for Angela, who you know has a learning disability. She is able to look after her own physical needs, but her family says that Angela has made some unwise decisions about her life that have resulted in her being 'taken advantage of'. Her family does not think that she is able to make decisions about her care. This information has been relayed to your team, and the team is therefore making care decisions without involving Angela.

Questions

- What does the law say about how Angela is being treated?
- Are these decisions right or wrong from a legal perspective?
- Has the decision about Angela's capacity to make choices about her care been properly made?

In such circumstances as in Box 2.4, the Mental Capacity Act of 2005 (see Chapter 5 for details) should be used as your guide, and this is the law that protects both Angela and you in your practice. This law would say that Angela is being treated unfairly, and such decisions made by her family are unlawful unless Angela has been properly assessed as lacking the competence to make such decisions. If consent is given by another person without legal capacity to consent being established, then the consent is not valid. You need to make sure that you advocate for Angela and facilitate the completion of the proper assessment of her capacity before you allow decisions about her care to be made for her.

Principles of consent have been recognised in case law for 100 years. In an early American case in which the wishes of the claimant, Mary Schloendorff, were ignored (*Schloendorff* v. *Society of New York Hospital* [1914]), the judge ruled that:

> *Every human being of adult years and sound mind has a right to determine what shall be done with his own body; and a surgeon who performs an operation without his patient's consent commits an assault for which he is liable in damages. This is true except in cases of emergency where the patient is unconscious and where it is necessary to operate before consent can be obtained.*
>
> (*Schloendorff* v. *Society of New York Hospital [1914]*)

The legal standard outlining the duty to inform patients about any risks or side effects was set in the case of *Sidaway* v. *Board of Governors of the Bethlem Royal Hospital* [1985] (see Box 2.5). It is necessary for you to explain any of the general risks to people in your care when gaining consent for any procedures or in administering medication, for example.

Box 2.5

Sidaway v. *Bethlem Royal Hospital Governors* [1985]

Amy Sidaway suffered from chronic persistent pain in her neck and shoulders. She was advised by her surgeon to have an operation near her spinal column to relieve the pain. The surgeon did not warn her of the less than 1% chance of damage to the spinal cord. During the surgery, the patient sustained damage to her spinal cord and was paralysed as a result. She was unable to claim damages because the surgery had been carried out correctly, but she sued for negligence on the basis that she had not been informed of all the risks.

In this case, the '*Bolam*' test (The test used to assess the appropriate standard of care: *Bolam* v. *Friern Hospital Management Committee* [1957] 1 WLR 582) (see Box 5.8) was applied, and it was found that a respectable body of opinion would not warn of such remote risks of this kind. Lord Templeton found that it is only necessary to give general risks in such cases.

In terms of gaining consent from children (those below the age of 16 years; DH 2009) and young people (those aged 16–17 years; DH 2009), the legal view is different to adults. According to the Family Law Act (1969), people aged 16–17 are presumed as having capacity to consent to their own medical treatment and related procedures, but if they refuse a treatment their decision can be overridden by a court or someone with parental responsibility (DH 2009). In assessing competence, the criteria used to assess adults should also be applied (DH 2009).

For children under the age of 16 years, the Gillick competence test can be applied. This is based on the case of *Gillick* v. *West Norfolk and Wisbech Area Health Authority* [1986] (see Box 2.6).

Box 2.6

Gillick v. *West Norfolk and Wisbech Area Health Authority* [1986]

In 1982, Mrs Victoria Gillick took her local health authority (West Norfolk and Wisbech Area Health Authority) and the DH and Social Security to court in an attempt to stop doctors from giving contraceptive advice or treatment to those under 16 years old without parental consent.

According to the Gillick case, under certain circumstances a child under the age of 16 could give valid consent without the involvement of their parent or guardian. The court found that a child below 16 years of age will be competent to consent to medical treatment if they have sufficient intelligence and understanding to understand what is proposed. Mr Justice Woolf concluded:

> *Whether or not a child is capable of giving the necessary consent will depend on the child's maturity and understanding and the nature of the consent required. The child must be capable of making a reasonable assessment of*

the advantages and disadvantages of the treatment proposed, so the consent, if given, can be properly and fairly described as true consent.

When commenting on the Gillick case in the House of Lords, Lord Scarman added:

It is not enough that she should understand the nature of the advice which is being given: she must also have a sufficient maturity to understand what is involved.

This test, often referred to as 'Gillick competence', is now used more widely to determine whether a child is able to consent. However, if a young person who has the capacity to consent or a Gillick-competent child refuses treatment, this refusal could be overturned if it is probable that the refusal would lead to death or severe permanent injury (DH 2009). If a child lacks the capacity to consent, consent can be given on their behalf under the 'welfare' or 'best interests' principle whilst involving the child as much as possible (DH 2009).

Consent in medical and nursing research

Consent to participate in medical or nursing research is also underpinned by governing principles. The historical development of these principles was born out of the atrocities that occurred during the Second World War, during which people were used as human subjects for experimentation without consent. The Nuremberg trials led to the development of the Nuremberg Code (1947). The judgement by the war crimes tribunal at Nuremberg laid down 10 standards to which physicians must conform when carrying out experiments on human subjects. The Declaration of Helsinki (1964) was further developed to safeguard people participating in biomedical research, medical research combined with professional care (clinical research) and non-therapeutic biomedical research involving human subjects.

Whilst as a student you may not be directly recruiting people into the types of research studies described previously, you can still advocate for those in your care and ensure that their interests are protected should they be recruited into such studies. You may be involved in such studies at some time in your career, particularly if you work as a research nurse or if you are planning to carry out your own research study.

The RCN (2009) published clear guidance on the conduct of research; this guidance includes the importance of informed consent. Some key points on informed consent from this guidance include the following:

- Consent should be obtained before entering or recruiting any participant into a research project.
- Participants should be fully informed of the research aims, potential benefits and harms.

- Consent must be voluntary; participants must not be coerced or unduly persuaded by rewards.
- Information about the study must be transparent and presented in a language that the participant can understand.
- Information should be given in verbal and written forms.
- Participants should be given sufficient time to consider their involvement and ask questions.
- Ideally, the consent form should be signed and witnessed, but this is not always required.
- Participants must be informed of their right to withdraw their consent to participate without this having an impact on their care.

Keeping clear and accurate records

Irving et al. (2006) suggested that much nursing documentation lacks structure and allows important information to be lost to the reader. In addition, it would seem that listening to a person in your care, teaching them and advocating for them are less likely to be documented (Hyde et al. 2005; Friberg et al. 2006), even though these skills are key to the provision of good care.

In March 2011, litigation in the NHS cost an estimated £16.6 billion as a result of clinical negligence claims (Furedi and Bristow 2012). The amount spent on damages and legal fees in 2010/2011 amounted to £768 million. In addition, the National Patient Safety Agency (2007) cited incomplete and inadequate documentation as a factor contributing to clinical deterioration. This includes decisions not being recorded in the patients' notes or discrepancies between what is recorded and what actually happened. Unsatisfactory documentation can also result in poor communication between professionals, which will result in compromised care (Health Service Ombudsman 2000).

There are many valid reasons for keeping clear and accurate records in nursing. These include the following:

- Demonstration of decision-making processes in care delivery;
- Support for communication between members of the multi-disciplinary team;
- Early identification of risks;
- Evidence when dealing with complaints, legal or safeguarding processes;
- Data for audit, research or service improvement;

- Documentation of delegated care;
- Evidence of care outcomes;
- Documentation of the patient journey;
- Improvement of quality of care.

The NMC (2009) provided clear guidance for record-keeping, which is summarised in Box 2.7.

Box 2.7

Guidance for record-keeping (summarised from NMC 2009)

Records should:

1. Be legible
2. Be signed, with your name and job title printed alongside the first entry
3. Be dated and timed in chronological order
4. Be accurate and clear
5. Be factual (without unnecessary abbreviations or jargon)
6. Be relevant (based on your professional judgement)
7. Include details of any assessments, reviews and plans for ongoing care
8. Identify any risks or problems and actions taken to deal with them
9. Be used to communicate fully and effectively with your colleagues
10. Not be altered or destroyed without authorisation
11. If necessary, be altered clearly and include the original entry
12. Include involvement from the person in your care or their carer
13. Include language that can be understood by the people in your care
14. Be readable when photocopied or scanned
15. Not include coded expressions of sarcasm or humorous abbreviations to describe the people in your care
16. Not be falsified

If the records are electronic, they must be traceable to the person who completed them. If record-keeping is delegated to a student or a healthcare support worker, the record should be countersigned by a registered nurse, who should decide if it is appropriate to delegate the task (RCN 2012).

Glasper (2011, p. 886) proposed a CIA mnemonic to remember when maintaining records. They should be

- **C**lear
- **I**ntelligible
- **A**ccurate

Glasper (2011, p. 887) further recommended the 'NO ELBOW' rule that may help you to develop your skills when completing paper records:

- No–**E**rasing
- No–**L**eaves (pages) pulled out or removed
- No–**B**lank spaces (draw a line across any blank spaces to avoid additions at a later stage)
- No–**O**verwriting
- No–**W**riting in margins

The one other key thing to remember is that everything you write could be read by the person to whom you are providing care. Therefore, you must not include emotive phrases or value judgements (Prideaux 2011). In addition, if any complaints are made or there is an action for negligence, all notes made that relate to the complainant (or their representative) will be scrutinised for what was written and for what was omitted. Think about your records as the evidence of what you do in your everyday work as a nurse.

Accountability

As a nurse you are personally accountable for your actions and your omissions in your practice, and you must always be able to justify your decisions; you are answerable for your actions and omissions even if you have been given instructions by another professional (NMC 2008). It is therefore necessary for you to carefully consider the actions you take (Tee 2009), particularly if a task or procedure is delegated to you. Some nurses think that accountability is about being blamed, but this defensive practice can result in an overreliance on protocols rather than the promotion of critical thinking and clinical judgement (Caulfield 2005).

You are accountable to

- Society through the public law;
- Patients through the law of negligence;
- Your employer through the law of contract;
- The nursing profession through the NMC.

Caulfield (2005) suggested that accountability is an inherent confidence that allows you as a nurse to take pride in being transparent about how you carry out your practice. Each time you justify your actions to others and document care delivery (or reasons for omissions) and outcome of care delivery, you are exercising your accountability (Hood 2013).

Caulfield (2005) provided a useful framework based on four pillars that will help you to understand and exercise your accountability. These pillars set out four types of authority in nursing: professional, ethical, legal and employment (Caulfield 2005, p. 3).

Professional accountability is based on the ethos that you promote the welfare and well-being of those in your care through the care that you deliver and therefore provides a framework for your practice (Caulfield 2005). The standards set by the NMC are the minimum requirements for your professional behaviour and practice. The NMC has clear expectations of you as a nurse, and the public should, through the NMC, trust that you are adhering to these standards. It is clear that the NMC sees you as responsible for your practice regardless of the influence of others.

Ethical accountability relates to your ethical values and provides the second pillar of accountability in your practice (Caulfield 2005). You had the opportunity to reflect on your own values in Chapter 1, and you will draw on your values when making and justifying care decisions. Your values may be questioned or challenged by situations in practice, so it is important to consider how those values have an impact on your accountability for your practice.

Legal accountability is underpinned by the laws governing your practice (key legislation is addressed in Chapter 5). Caulfield (2005) suggested that nurses are not always conversant with the law governing their practice and are therefore unclear about how the law has an impact on them as practitioners. You should not be fearful of the law; it is not only there to protect those in your care but is also there to protect and guide you and help you to justify your practice.

Employment accountability relates to the contract you have with your employing organisation. When employed, you will have a contract of employment detailing the relationship you have with your employer and the agreed role and responsibilities you will be accountable for (Caulfield 2005). The contract will also define the systems within which you will be expected to work. Your contract should be clear because the organisation is vicariously liable for your practice (i.e. if you do something wrong and a person in your care is harmed as a result of your acts or omissions, your employing organisation will be liable to pay damages). You should be aware that if you work outside these agreed roles and responsibilities without prior agreement, or not attend mandatory training as expected, for example, this may negate the support provided to you through your employment contract.

Accountability is essential in protecting people who receive care and treatment (Griffith 2013).

Delegation of duties

The National Leadership and Innovations Agency for Healthcare (2010, p. 3) developed a useful definition of delegation as

> *the process by which you (the delegator) allocate clinical or non-clinical treatment or care to a competent person (the delegatee). You will remain responsible for the overall management of the service user, and accountable for your decision to delegate. You will not be accountable for the decisions and actions of the delegatee.*

Delegation of duties links closely with accountability. As a student, you will regularly have care delivery or procedures delegated to you. You have a duty of care, and you are therefore legally liable should your acts or omissions result in harm. If a procedure or form of care delivery is delegated to you, you must perform it competently. If you do not feel competent to carry out the delegated task, or if you believe the delegation of the task goes against agreed protocols or procedures, you are responsible for saying so.

The RCN (2010) suggested that for someone to be accountable they must

- Have the ability to perform the task,
- Accept the responsibility for doing the task, and
- Have the authority to perform the task within their job description and the policies and protocols of the organisation.

The National Leadership and Innovations Agency for Healthcare (2010, p. 10) identified questions that should be asked about the task:

- **Can the task be delegated?** Here, the level of the task should be taken into account, as should the skills the individual would need to perform the task. Does the task need to be delegated?
- **Can this task only be performed by a registered professional?** Consider whether the task must be performed by someone in a particular profession.
- **Do the benefits outweigh the risk to the service user?** The benefits of delegating the task should outweigh the risks.
- **Do you need to gain service user consent?**
- **Have you gained service user consent?** Have you consulted with the service user and made them aware that the task being undertaken on them will be conducted by an identified individual?

When considering the delegation of a task, registered nurses must ensure that the task is delegated appropriately (RCN 2010). The following guidance refers to support workers, but it also applies to students:

- The task is necessary, and delegation is in the patient's best interest.
- The support worker understands the task and how it is to be performed.
- The support worker has the skills and abilities to perform the task competently.
- The support worker accepts the responsibility to perform the task competently.

Now, read the scenario in Box 2.8 and use this section's information to form a response.

Box 2.8

Practice scenario: accountability and responsibility

You are currently in a practice placement, and one of the registered nurses, John, asks you to administer some medication. John says that he is happy for you to do this whilst he gives medication to someone else. You question if you should be doing it alone, and John says that he is confident that you can do it unsupervised because he observed you doing it before and you did it correctly last time.

- What would you do in this situation and why?

This scenario is common and can be a difficult one for you particularly when you are trying to demonstrate your skills, ability to work independently and willingness to participate in all aspects of care. However, when a medication chart is signed by a registered nurse, that nurse is signing to indicate that he or she has dispensed the medication and has witnessed that it was taken or administered. This therefore is not really a question of your ability, but a legal requirement. The registered nurse is accountable for ensuring that the medication is given to the correct person and is therefore accountable for any delegation. The registered nurse should not delegate this responsibility to you unless he or she is observing you directly. John should be observing you in such circumstances. You could respond to John by saying that you are happy to take on all aspects of the task but politely ask that he observe you. Remember that as a student you are not allowed to accept responsibility for anything that is outside your sphere of competence; administering medication unsupervised is outside your sphere of competence as a student nurse because you are not yet a qualified nurse.

Chapter summary

The way in which you practise is fundamentally underpinned by your professional code and by requirements set by the NMC. This chapter introduced the NMC as your professional governing body. The purpose of the NMC was summarised, and you were introduced to your professional code. You had the opportunity to explore the concepts of confidentiality, consent, record-keeping, accountability and delegation and consider how they relate to your practice. Being a professional nurse is complex, but the NMC, other organisations such as the RCN and the law are there to help you circumnavigate these complexities so that you can deliver high standards of safe and effective care and justify the care decisions you make on a day-to-day basis.

References

Bolam v. *Friern Hospital Management Committee* [1957] 1 WLR 582.

Buka, P. 2008. *Patients' Rights, Law and Ethics for Nurses: A Practical Guide* London: Hodder Arnold.

Caulfield, H. 2005. *Accountability: Vital Notes for Nurses*. Oxford, UK: Blackwell.

Data Protection Act. 1998. Available from: http://www.legislation.gov.uk/ukpga/1998/29/contents (accessed 17 October 2013).

Declaration of Helsinki 1964. *British Medical Journal* 1996; 313: 1148.2

Department of Health (DH). 1997. *The Caldicott Committee Report on the Review of Patient-Identifiable Information*. Available from: http://webarchive.nationalarchives.gov.uk/20130107105354/http://www.dh.gov.uk/prod_consum_dh/groups/dh_digitalassets/@dh/@en/documents/digitalasset/dh_4068404.pdf (accessed 17 October 2013).

Department of Health (DH). 2003. *Confidentiality: NHS Code of Practice*. London: Department of Health. Available from: https://www.gov.uk/government/uploads/system/uploads/attachment_data/file/200146/Confidentiality_-_NHS_Code_of_Practice.pdf (accessed 17 October 2013).

Department of Health (DH). 2009. *Reference Guide to Consent for Examination or Treatment*. 2nd edn. London: Department of Health. Available from: https://www.gov.uk/government/publications/reference-guide-to-consent-for-examination-or-treatment-second-edition (accessed 17 October 2013).

Department of Health (DH). 2013. *Information: To Share or Not to Share, Government Response to the Caldicott Review*. Available from: https://www.gov.uk/government/uploads/system/uploads/attachment_data/file/239273/9731-2901141-TSO-Caldicott-Government_Response_ACCESSIBLE.pdf (accessed 17 October 2013).

Friberg. F., Bergh, A., Lepp, M. 2006. In search of details of patient teaching in nursing documentation—an analysis of patient records in a medical ward in Sweden. *Journal of Clinical Nursing* 15(12): 1550–1558.

Furedi, F., Bristow, J. 2012. *The Social Cost of Litigation*. Chichester, UK: Centre for Policy Studies.

Gillick v. *West Norfolk and Wisbech Area Health Authority* [1986] 3 All ER 492.

Glasper, A. 2011. Improving record keeping: Important lessons for nurses. *British Journal of Nursing* 20(14): 886–887.

Griffith, R. 2013. Nurse-led clinics: Accountability and practice. *Nurse Prescribing* 11(4): 196–199.

Health Service Ombudsman. 2000. *Fifth Report for Session 1999–2000. Selected Cases and Summaries of Completed Investigations October 1999–March 2000*. London: Stationery Office.

Hood, L.J. 2013. *Leddy and Pepper's Conceptual Bases of Professional Nursing* (8th Edn). Philadelphia: Lippincott Williams and Wilkins.

Human Fertilisation and Embryology Act. 2008. Great Britain. Available from: http://www.legislation.gov.uk/ukpga/2008/22/contents (accessed 18 December 2013).

Human Rights Act. 1998. Available from: http://www.legislation.gov.uk/ukpga/1998/42/introduction (accessed 17 October 2013).

Hyde, A., Treacy, M., Scott, A., et al. 2005. Modes of rationality in nursing documentation: Biology, biography and the 'voice of nursing'. *Nursing Inquiry* 12(2): 66–68.

Irving, K., Treacy, M., Scott, A., Hyde, A., Butler, M., MacNeela, P. 2006. Discursive practices in the documentation of patient assessments. *Journal of Advanced Nursing* 53(2): 151–159.

Mental Capacity Act. 2005. Available from: http://www.legislation.gov.uk/ukpga/2005/9/section/22 (accessed 17 October 2013).

National Leadership and Innovations Agency for Healthcare. 2010. *All Wales Guidelines for Delegation*. Available from: http://www.wales.nhs.uk/sitesplus/documents/829/All%20Wales%20Guidelines%20for%20Delegation.pdf (accessed 19 November 2013).

National Patient Safety Agency. 2007. *Recognising and Responding Appropriately to Early Signs of Deterioration in Hospitalised Patients*. Available from: http://www.nrls.npsa.nhs.uk/resources/?entryid45=59834 (accessed 17 October 2013).

Nursing and Midwifery Council (NMC). 2001. Nursing and Midwifery order Available from: http://www.legislation.gov.uk/uksi/2002/253/contents/made (accessed 26 April 2014).

Nursing and Midwifery Council (NMC). 2008. *The Code: Standards of Conduct, Performance and Ethics for Nurses and Midwives*. London: NMC.

Nursing and Midwifery Council (NMC). 2009. *Record Keeping. Guidance for Nurses and Midwives.* London: NMC. Available from: http://www.nmc-uk.org/Documents/NMC-Publications/NMC-Record-Keeping-Guidance.pdf (accessed 17 October 2013).

Nursing and Midwifery Council (NMC). 2011. *Guidance on Professional Conduct for Nursing and Midwifery Students.* Available from: http://www.nmc-uk.org/Documents/NMC-Publications/NMC-Guidance-on-professional-conduct.pdf (accessed 17 October 2013).

Nursing and Midwifery Council (NMC). 2013. *Consent.* Available from: http://www.nmc-uk.org/Nurses-and-midwives/Regulation-in-practice/Regulation-in-Practice-Topics/consent/ (accessed 2 January 2014).

Prideaux, A. 2011. Issues in nursing documentation and record-keeping practice. *British Journal of Nursing* 20(22): 1450–1454.

Royal College of Nursing (RCN). 2009. *Research Ethics. Guidance for Nurses.* London: RCN. Available from: http://www.rcn.org.uk/__data/assets/pdf_file/0007/388591/003138.pdf (accessed 17 October 2013).

Royal College of Nursing. 2010. *Accountability and Delegation: What You Need to Know.* https://www.rcn.org.uk/__data/assets/pdf_file/0003/381720/003942.pdf (accessed 19 November 2013).

Royal College of Nursing (RCN). 2012. *Record Keeping—The Facts.* Available from: http://www.rcn.org.uk/__data/assets/pdf_file/0005/476753/Record_keeping_cards_V5.pdf (accessed 17 October 2013).

R v. *Department of Health ex parte Source Informatics Ltd.* [2001] QB 424; [2000] 2 WLR 940; [2000] 1 All ER 786.

Schloendorff v. *Society of New York Hospital* [1914] 211 N.Y. 125; 105 N.E. 92; 1914 N.Y.

Sidaway *v.* Bethlem Royal Hospital Governors [1985] 1 All ER 643.

Tee, S.R. 2009. Ethical and legal principles for health care. In Childs, L.L., Coles, L., and Marjoram, B. (eds.), *Essential Skills Clusters for Nurses: Theory for Practice.* West Sussex, UK: Wiley-Blackwell, 121–140.

The Nuremberg Code 1947. *BMJ* 1996; 313: 1448.1 Available from: www.bmj.com/content/313/7070/1448.1 (accessed 26 April 2014).

W v. *Egdell* [1990] 1 All ER 835.

3

Expectations of professional nurses

Introduction

This chapter provides an exploration of the expectations of a nurse from broad perspectives, including the media image of nursing, what the public and patient groups expect from nurses providing care, National Health Service (NHS) expectations of registered nurses and standards of public life. High-profile public inquiries relevant to the image of nursing are explored in relation to the provision of safe and quality care and the public image of nursing. The need to treat people as individuals and inspire their trust is discussed. The elements of fitness to practise, including good character, are explained to allow you to reflect on your behaviour and image as a professional nurse.

Learning outcomes

By the end of this chapter, you will be able to

- Explain the relationship between public expectations of you as a nurse and quality and safety in nursing practice;
- Appreciate the concept of good character in relation to professional nursing practice;
- Uphold and promote a positive image of nursing;
- Reflect on self- and possible public perceptions of your behaviour as a nurse.

The NHS Constitution

The NHS Constitution (Department of Health [DH] 2013) sets out the principles and values of the NHS in England, more specifically,

> *rights to which patients, public and staff are entitled, and pledges which the NHS is committed to achieve, together with responsibilities, which the public, patients and staff owe to one another to ensure that the NHS operates fairly and effectively.*
>
> *(p. 2)*

The constitution sets the legal requirement for all NHS bodies, private and voluntary sector providers supplying NHS services and local authorities to apply the constitution when making decisions and taking action. The NHS Constitution is underpinned by seven principles (see Box 3.1).

Box 3.1

The NHS Constitution: seven underpinning principles (DH 2013)*

1. The NHS provides a **comprehensive service**, available to all irrespective of gender, race, disability, age, sexual orientation, religion, belief, gender reassignment, pregnancy and maternity or marital or civil partnership status.
2. Access to NHS services is based on **clinical need**, not an individual's ability to pay.
3. The NHS aspires to the **highest standards** of excellence and professionalism.
4. The NHS aspires to put **patients** at the heart of everything it does.
5. The NHS works across organisational boundaries and in **partnership** with other organisations in the interest of patients, local communities and the wider population.
6. The NHS is committed to providing **best value** for taxpayers' money and the most effective, fair and sustainable use of finite resources. Public funds for health care will be devoted solely to the benefit of the people that the NHS serves.
7. The NHS is **accountable** to the public, communities and patients that it serves.

* Department of Health. 2013. *The NHS Constitution for England*. Available from: https://www.gov.uk/government/publications/the-nhsconstitution-for-england (accessed 24 November 2013).

The NHS Constitution also details rights afforded to patients, to the public and to you as an NHS employee. In helping you to provide a professional standard of care in a safe, high-quality environment, the NHS commits to

- Providing you with a positive working environment and promotes supportive, open cultures that help you do your job to the best of your ability;
- Providing you with clear roles and responsibilities and rewarding jobs that make a difference to patients, their families and carers and communities;
- Providing you with personal development, access to appropriate education and training, and line management support;
- Providing you with support and opportunities for you to maintain your health, well-being and safety;

- Engaging you in decisions that affect you and the services you provide;
- Having a process for you to raise an internal grievance;
- Encouraging and supporting you in raising concerns at the earliest reasonable opportunity about safety, malpractice or wrongdoing at work.

In return for this commitment to you, through the NHS Constitution (as well as your own professional body), you are required to practise with the values detailed in the constitution. These core values (also mentioned in Chapter 1) were developed in consultation with patients, public and staff to 'inspire passion in the NHS':

- Working together for patients
- Respect and dignity
- Commitment to quality of care
- Compassion
- Improving lives
- Everyone counts

In addition, you have a duty

- To accept professional accountability and maintain the standards of professional practice;
- To take reasonable care of health and safety at work for you, your team and others and to cooperate with employers to ensure compliance with health and safety requirements;
- To act in accordance with the express and implied terms of your contract of employment;
- Not to discriminate against patients or staff and to adhere to equal opportunities and equality and human rights legislation;
- To protect the confidentiality of personal information that you hold;
- To be honest and truthful in applying for a job and in carrying out that job.

Activity

Reflecting on your everyday practice, what **behaviours** do you exhibit on a daily basis to take responsibility for your own health and safety and that of your team? Think of behaviours that do not involve people in your care, but think specifically about your own safety and that of your colleagues. These behaviours can be related to anything from arriving for your shift on time to carrying out risk assessments on equipment, for example.

Standards in public life

The Committee on Standards in Public Life is an independent public body that provides advice to the government on ethical standards in public life in the United Kingdom (http://www.public-standards.gov.uk/). The committee was established in 1994 amid concerns about greater scrutiny of the conduct of people in public positions and the media response to misconduct in public life. Whilst it was generally recognised that most people in public positions met the expectations of the public, weakness in enforcing and maintaining the standards were identified, as were concerns about the boundaries of acceptable conduct befitting those in public positions (Nolan 1995). In what became known as the Nolan Report, the committee proposed Seven Principles of Public Life: selflessness, integrity, objectivity, accountability, openness, honesty and leadership. These principles applied to people elected or appointed to public office, as a civil servant, to work in local government; in the police, courts and probation services; and in health, education, social and care services; and those delivering public services. In addition, the report made 55 specific recommendations for members of Parliament, civil servants, public bodies and NHS bodies. In summarising these, the committee recommended that all public bodies incorporate the seven principles into their codes of conduct, that there should be independent scrutiny of how the standards are maintained, and that there should be more investment in promoting and reinforcing the standards through guidance and education.

In 2013, the Committee on Standards in Public Life (2013) produced its 14th report regarding the outcomes of a review of best practice in promoting good behaviour in public life. Whilst this report does apply to all public life and organisations, there are some stark lessons for health care and nursing. Despite the introduction of the Seven Principles of Public Life, which are reviewed in this 2013 report (see Table 3.1), the committee has grave concerns about failings in public organisations, including within the NHS, and doubts about the behaviours of some of the people working within those organisations, including nurses (see the discussion of the review into Mid Staffordshire NHS Trust and the Keogh review that follows in this chapter). Whilst progress with the Seven Principles of Public Life has been made, there is clear evidence that there is still work to do in ensuring that these principles are embedded, monitored and maintained.

Activity

Reflect on your professional code and on your own values and behaviours.

How do the principles of public life (Table 3.1) reflect your own nursing practice?

Table 3.1 The Seven Principles of Public Life

Principle	Revised description
Selflessness	Holders of public office should act solely in terms of the public interest.
Integrity	Holders of public office must avoid placing themselves under any obligation to people or organisations that might try inappropriately to influence them in their work. They should not act or take decisions to gain financial or other material benefits for themselves, their family, or their friends. They must declare and resolve any interests and relationships.
Objectivity	Holders of public office must act and take decisions impartially, fairly and on merit, using the best evidence and without discrimination or bias.
Accountability	Holders of public office are accountable to the public for their decisions and actions and must submit themselves to the scrutiny necessary to ensure this.
Openness	Holders of public office should act and take decisions in an open and transparent manner. Information should not be withheld from the public unless there are clear and lawful reasons for so doing.
Honesty	Holders of public office should be truthful.
Leadership	Holders of public office should exhibit these principles in their own behaviour. They should actively promote and robustly support the principles and be willing to challenge poor behaviour wherever it occurs.

Source: Committee on Standards in Public Life. 2013. *Standards Matter. A Review of Best Practice in Promoting Good Behaviour in Public Life. Fourteenth Report of the Committee on Standards in Public Life.* London: HMSO. Available from: http:// www.public-standards.gov.uk/wp-content/uploads/2013/01/Standards_Matter.pdf (accessed 10 December 2013).

Media influence on the public image of nursing

Virginia Henderson (1978) suggested that the self-image of nurses and what nurses do is often at odds with the public's image of nursing and what the public thinks nurses do. It would seem that this discourse remains prevalent today, with the public image of nurses not always matching their professional image (Ten Hoeve et al. 2013). This is not helped by the stereotypes that continue to be formed in the media, and these continue to reflect the four images of nursing identified by Bridges (1990) of the ministering angel, the battleaxe, the naughty nurse and the doctor's handmaiden. For example, the public do not always appreciate the fact that nurses are well educated (Summers and Summers 2009) or necessarily recognise the scientific and professional development of the nursing profession (Ten Hoeve et al. 2013) because of the regular negative images of nursing presented in the media. Ten Hoeve et al. (2013) suggested that the public image of nursing is predominantly based on misconceptions and stereotypes resulting from distorted images of nurses in the media.

The viewing public 'seem to hold an endless fascination' (Jackson 2009, p. 2249) with hospitals. Czarny et al. (2008) found that most nursing students watch television, with medical dramas common in their viewing, and that the images and messages in these television programmes can form a part of the informal curriculum. Nurses continue to be the focus of television shows, documentaries and advertising; this is because of the array of characters and scenarios that can be explored (Weaver et al. 2013). Weaver et al. therefore carried out a study to explore nursing students' perceptions of their profession on television. They found that the general public's views about the nursing profession are influenced heavily by the representation of nursing on television, and that the negative portrayal of nursing can create a false image of the profession. Weaver et al. found that nursing students view the images of nursing seen on television as misleading and incorrect and made for poor role models because of the negative stereotyping depicted in the television roles. They concluded by confirming that the images of the doctor's handmaiden and the sex symbol continue to be propagated by the media. They suggested that students want a more 'visible, accurate and realistic' portrayal of nursing represented on television so that the general public are more informed of the skilled, intelligent and assertive modern nurse working in health care today (Weaver et al. 2013). Weaver et al. concluded that images of nursing displayed in the media can shape, reinforce or develop nursing stereotypes, and this can damage the value and status of the nursing profession. Cabaniss (2011) also suggested that a positive image of nursing is important in recruiting the right students to the nursing profession.

It would seem that the image of nurses in the media falls short of the professional image of nursing (Ten Hoeve et al. 2013). Ten Hoeve et al. suggested that nurses need to work to improve the public image of the nursing profession by raising awareness of what nurses actually do, the different roles available in nursing, and the qualifications they need to gain to register and practise. Fletcher (2007) suggested that as individual nurses work to enhance their own professional image, the public image of nursing will reflect this.

Activity

Visit YouTube and search for 'nurse image'. Select a few of the films that portray negative images of nursing and positive images of nursing.

- What stereotypes of nurses still exist? Consider 'stereotype' as an impression of a group that people form by associating particular characteristics and emotions with that group (Smith and Mackie 2007).
- What are your feelings about the way nursing is portrayed? How does this affect the way in which you view your chosen profession?

Public inquiries and their impact on images of nursing

In 2013, reports from two highly publicised inquiries were published. Both of these have important implications for nursing as a profession and public images of nurses.

Mid Staffordshire NHS Foundation Trust Public Inquiry

Between January 2005 and March 2009, it was estimated that 400–1,200 people died as a result of poor care at Stafford Hospital, part of Mid Staffordshire NHS Hospital Foundation Trust. In June 2010, the then-Secretary of State for Health Andrew Lansley announced that there would be a public inquiry into the high rates of deaths. Between November 2010 and December 2011, the inquiry heard 352 witness statements from patients, hospital staff, board members, ministers and senior civil servants. The inquiry also included seven public seminars and seven fact-finding visits to various healthcare organisations. The remit of the inquiry was to establish what was done by the commissioning, supervisory and regulatory bodies (including the Care Quality Commission, the Health and Safety Executive, local scrutiny and public engagement bodies and the local coroner) and systems in the NHS to identify poor care at Stafford Hospital, what they did about it, and why something had not been done sooner. More than a million pages of evidence were produced, and the cost of the inquiry at November 2013 was an estimated £13 million.

Francis (2013) cited a catalogue of failings in the care of patients, which resulted in preventable suffering. Examples included the following:

- Basic elements of care were neglected.
- Patients needed pain relief and received it late or not at all.
- Patients were left unwashed for up to a month.
- Food and drinks were left out of the reach of patients.
- Many patients had to rely on family members for help with feeding.
- Patients were sent home before they should have been, resulting in an unnecessary readmission to the hospital.
- Hygiene standards were poor to the extent that some families were removing used dressings from public areas and were cleaning toilets.

- Patients were left in soiled beds or left sitting on a commode after calls for help were ignored.
- Patients were commonly misdiagnosed.

Activity

- What media coverage was there of the failings at Stafford Hospital?
- What impact do you think the Francis Inquiry and report had on the public image of nursing? Was it damaging to the nursing profession, and if so, why?

People expected to be cared for, but instead a whole system failed them, a system that ignored the early warning signs that problems existed and put corporate needs and cost saving before the needs of patients. Whilst this public inquiry focussed on one NHS trust, there was sufficient evidence to cast doubt on practices across the NHS as a whole. The outcomes of this inquiry had far-reaching consequences for the entire NHS and, in fact, the nursing profession. Francis (2013) made a total of 290 recommendations, summarised by the following (Francis 2013, pp. 4–5):

- Foster a common culture shared by all in the service of putting the patient first.
- Develop a set of fundamental standards, easily understood and accepted by patients, the public and healthcare staff, the breach of which should not be tolerated.
- Provide professionally endorsed and evidence-based means of compliance with these fundamental standards which can be understood and adopted by the staff who have to provide the service.
- Ensure openness, transparency and candour throughout the system about matters of concern.
- Ensure that the relentless focus of the healthcare regulator is on policing compliance with these standards.
- Make all those who provide patient care—individuals and organisations—properly accountable for what they do and ensure that the public is protected from those not fit to provide such a service.
- Provide for a proper degree of accountability for senior managers and leaders to place all with responsibility for protecting the interests of patients on a level playing field.
- Enhance the recruitment, education, training and support of all the key contributors to the provision of health care, but in particular those in nursing and leadership positions, to integrate the essential shared values of the common culture into everything they do.

Activity

In considering the nursing contribution to the failings at the trust, Francis (2013) was clear that there should be an increased focus on caring, compassionate and considerate nursing in the education of nurses in pre-registration and across post-registration education.

- Thinking about what you have read in Chapters 1 and 2, and in light of the failings in care alluded to regarding the Stafford Hospital, do you think these aspects of nursing have been lost, and if so, why?
- Do you consider yourself to be a caring, compassionate and considerate nurse, and what does this mean to you?
- How would you work to prevent such failings from occurring in the future?

- Develop and share ever-improving means of measuring and understanding the performance of individual professionals, teams, units and provider organisations for the patients, the public, and all other stakeholders in the system.

The Keogh mortality review

On 6 February 2013, Professor Sir Bruce Keogh, NHS medical director for England, was asked by the prime minister to carry out a review into the quality of care and treatment provided by NHS trusts and NHS foundation trusts that had higher-than-average mortality rates. The investigation looked at 14 organisations that had been selected using the mortality rate indicators. These indicators were used as a warning sign; therefore, the organisations were closely scrutinised for the following:

- **Mortality rates**
- **Patient experience**: understanding how the views of patients and related patient experience data are used and acted on
- **Safety**: understanding issues concerning the trust's safety record and ability to manage these issues
- **Workforce**: understanding issues regarding the trust's workforce and its strategy to deal with issues within the workforce as well as listening to the views of staff
- **Clinical and operational effectiveness**: understanding issues concerning the trust's clinical and operational performance, in particular how trusts use mortality data to analyse and improve quality of care
- **Governance and leadership**: understanding the trust's leadership and governance of quality

These indicators were identified as the core foundations of quality care.

It is interesting to note that the review was not scathing about individual nurses and the care delivered, but the report did highlight significant failings from a management and organisational perspective. Video of Sir Bruce Keogh talking about the review is available online (http://www.telegraph.co.uk/health/10183594/NHS-inquiry-Sir-Bruce-Keogh-disappointed-with-report-findings.html).

Concerns specific to nursing included concerns about levels of supervision, staffing numbers, numbers of nurses leaving the organisations, numbers of nurses joining the organisations and the difficulties nurses often had in referring patients to appropriate ongoing care. In summarising, Keogh (2013) actively encouraged directors of nursing to consider how they could make the most of the 'loyalty and innovation of student nurses, who move from ward to ward, so they become ambassadors for their hospital and for promoting innovative nursing practice' (p. 12).

Activity

Visit the BBC News website and watch the video 'Bedford Nurse Hits Back at Negative Image' (http://www.bbc.co.uk/news/uk-england-beds-bucks-herts-16759459).

- What are the key messages from this short news clip in relation to the public image of nursing?
- What can you do to improve the image of nursing in your everyday practice?
- Make note of your strategy but make sure this is realistic so that you can revisit it in 6 months to see if you have achieved it.

Public expectations and feedback

People expect to be treated with dignity and respect, and your Nursing and Midwifery Council (NMC) Code (NMC 2008, p. 2) states that you must treat people as individuals and respect their dignity (for a detailed discussion of dignity, see Chapter 6). People are different in many ways; therefore, they need to be treated as individuals. For example, whilst a diagnosis of a mental health disorder may be similar in nature when given to a number of individuals, people react in different ways to different situations. Their values, beliefs, backgrounds, and social, economic and religious positions can have an impact on how they deal with their illness, so these need to be taken into account. We are all different, which means people should expect that you, as a nurse, would respect these differences. It is necessary for you to design care that meets the needs of individuals at a particular point in time by learning about a person in your care and then modifying the care you deliver based on the person's wishes, needs and abilities (Radwin and Alster 2002).

You may find it difficult to deliver individualised care in some areas where standardised care pathways or care plans are used or where routines or task-orientated care govern care provision. However, reflect on your own expectations about care: How would you feel if care delivered did not meet your individual needs, or if you were not involved in your own care decisions? Standardisation of care should always be questioned and care tailored to each individual. Providing individualised care can have a positive impact on a person's experience of care (Suhonen et al. 2012), as highlighted in the document *Putting Patients First*, which assures commitment to ensuring that patients are at the centre of all care delivery and to increasing the patient voice (NHS England 2013). Chapter 7 focusses in detail on person-centred approaches to care.

The patient voice is essential in improving nursing care delivery, and you can see the impact of this in the Francis report discussed previously. In developing any professional requirements, guidance or standards, the NMC consults extensively with the public to ensure that their expectations are respected. The Code, for example, not only stipulates the standards expected of you but can also be used by the public to inform their expectations of you so that they can be confident in the care you deliver to them. The Standards for Pre-registration nursing education (NMC 2010), one of the domains of which underpins the development of this book, are also a result of extensive consultation with the public.

The public involvement in NMC work continues to increase through different forums, for example, the Patient Engagement Forum. The voice of the public has a strong influence on the nursing profession, and the public's views are noted. However, the feedback from the public does not always make for happy reading. In one Patient Engagement Forum facilitated by the NMC (NMC 2012), patient representatives from a variety of organisations suggested that nurses have lost the ethos of compassionate care and empathy and that dignity should be inherent because nurses should be treating people according to the Code. They further advised that nurses not only should be proud of their profession and want to know other colleagues are safe and competent, but also should be more accountable and responsible in raising concerns about their organisations or colleagues.

There have also been increased efforts within healthcare organisations generally to harness feedback from people receiving care so that improvements can be made. NHS Surveys (see http://www.nhssurveys.org/) carry out NHS patient surveys focussing on the patient experience. This programme is intended to systematically gather the view of patients about their recent care experiences. The surveys not only facilitate the development of a national picture of people's experiences of health care in the NHS but also help organisations make improvements to the services offered.

Activity

It is really important that you obtain feedback from those in your care about their experience of the care you are delivering. You should not, however, come across in a threatening manner. You must be able to take their feedback on board. Look at the number of ways in which feedback is gathered from service users and families in your workplace.

- How is feedback gathered and by whom?
- What is done with this feedback, and how does it influence the care delivered in your workplace?
- What can people in your care expect from the service you deliver? Is this articulated anywhere?

Fitness to practise

The public expects that you will be fit to practise throughout your career. The NMC describes fitness to practise as a person's suitability to be on the register without restrictions. Being fit to practise means that you have the skills, knowledge, good health and good character to do your job safely and effectively by adhering to principles of good practice set out by the NMC in standards, guidance and advice. However, it is about not only your professional performance but but also anything you do that might have an impact on public safety or confidence in the nursing profession. The expectations of your conduct and behaviour apply not only to your professional life but also how you conduct yourself in your personal life. Once you join the nursing profession, you are representing the profession both inside and outside your work environment. The NMC defined the conditions that constitute being unfit to practise as follows:

- **Misconduct**: behaviour that falls short of what is expected of a nurse
- **Lack of competence**: lack of knowledge, skill, performance or judgement
- **Character issues**: usually relating to criminal behaviour (e.g. a conviction or caution)
- **Poor health**: long-term serious physical or mental health conditions
- **Previous finding**: a finding by any other health or social care regulator or licensing body that a nurse or midwife's fitness to practise is impaired
- **Barring**: under the arrangements provided by the Safeguarding Vulnerable Groups Act of 2006, the Safeguarding Vulnerable Groups

(Northern Ireland) order of 2007 or the Protection of Vulnerable Groups (Scotland) Act of 2007

As highlighted in Chapter 2, the primary purpose of the NMC is public protection. It is therefore the NMC that, on the public's behalf, would make a judgement should your fitness to practise be called into question. If the NMC receives a complaint, the complaint will be referred to an investigating committee who will decide if there is a case to answer. The investigating committee can

- Close the case with no further action taken;
- Refer the case for an interim orders hearing;
- Refer the case to another investigating committee panel;
- Refer the case to the Conduct and Competence Committee; or
- Refer the case to a panel of the Health Committee.

The outcomes of NMC hearings are published on the NMC website (http://www.nmc-uk.org/Hearings/Hearings-and-outcomes/).

Good character

Being of good character relates to your conduct, behaviour and attitude as a professional nurse. Your character must be of a high calibre if you are to provide safe and quality care in practice. Everything you do must be compatible with your professional registration; if you engage in any behaviour that is not compatible, then your fitness to practise can be called into question. Usually, convictions, cautions and pending police charges are the more obvious reasons for questionable character, but a variety of behaviours and attitudes that are also unacceptable are demonstrated by some registered nurses. It is worth noting that you will be viewed as of a more favourable character if you disclose any previous convictions, cautions or pending police charges than if you try to conceal these criminal behaviours. Trying to hide such criminal wrongdoings is deceitful and is not compatible with being a registered nurse. As a student nurse, you are duty bound to report any convictions, cautions and pending police charges to your university before starting your course and at any time during the course should they arise. If you are unsure about what to report, you are advised to discuss it with one of your lecturers and the lecturer will be able to advise you.

The public need to know that you are honest in both your professional and personal life, and this includes your conduct as a student. The NMC (NMC 2011b) is clear about your conduct as a student. The conditions under which concern can be raised in relation to your conduct and behaviour are summarised in Table 3.2. Consider the practice scenario in Box 3.2 and the questions raised.

Table 3.2 Areas of Concern for Fitness to Practise in Nursing Students

Aggressive, violent or threatening behaviour	• Verbal, physical or mental abuse • Assault • Bullying • Physical violence
Cheating or plagiarising	• Cheating in examinations, coursework, clinical assessment or record books • Forging a mentor or tutor's name or signature on clinical assessments or record books • Passing off other people's work as your own
Criminal conviction or caution	• Child abuse or any other abuse • Child pornography • Fraud • Physical violence • Possession of illegal substance • Theft
Dishonesty	• Fraudulent curriculum vitae, application forms or other documents • Misrepresentation of qualifications
Drug or alcohol misuse	• Alcohol consumption that affects work • Dealing, possessing or misusing drugs • Drunk driving
Health concerns	• Failure to seek medical treatment or other support if there is a risk of harm to other people • Failure to recognise limits and abilities or lack of insight into health concerns that may put other people at risk
Persistent inappropriate attitude or behaviour	• Failure to accept and follow advice from your university or clinical placement provider • Non-attendance—clinical and academic • Poor application and failure to submit work • Poor communication skills
Unprofessional behaviour	• Breach of confidentiality • Misuse of the Internet and social networking sites • Failure to keep appropriate professional or sexual boundaries • Persistent rudeness to people, colleagues or others • Unlawful discrimination

Source: Nursing and Midwifery Council (NMC). 2011. *Guidance on Professional Conduct for Nursing and Midwifery Students.* Available from: http://www.nmc-uk.org/Documents/NMC-Publications/NMC-Guidance-on-professional-conduct.pdf (accessed 17 October 2013).

Box 3.2

Practice scenario: maintaining professional boundaries

You are working in an inpatient environment, and you notice that your friend Doreen is becoming over-familiar with Richard, who is under her care. You choose not to make an issue about it, but as the weeks progress you notice that this is becoming increasingly obvious. You discuss this with your mentor, who then meets with Doreen to remind her about maintaining professional boundaries, and she discusses the implications of forming inappropriate relationships with people in her care.

Later that month, Doreen shares some photos of an intimate nature with you, and you notice that Richard is the subject of these photos, which have also been posted on a social networking site. It becomes obvious to you that Doreen is now in a relationship with Richard, who has been transferred to the community team in which Doreen is working.

Questions

What, if anything, would you do with this information? If you did report it, what would your reasons be for doing so? What are the implications of reporting this for

1. Doreen?
2. Richard?
3. You?

The consequences for Doreen in Box 3.2 might be that she is disciplined or discontinued from the course, but this decision would be made in partnership with the relevant NHS trust or organisation within which this relationship occurred. You may feel that you have let your friend down or breached her confidence, but ultimately it is Richard's welfare that should be the focus of any action. When you are faced with such dilemmas, you need to consider who is most at risk or who is most vulnerable. Chapter 10 focusses on safeguarding in more detail, but it is really important that you discuss such concerns with one of your lecturers or your mentor if you encounter such situations in practice.

Integrity

Having integrity is an essential component of good character and is a desirable quality in you as a nurse. Laabs (2011) described integrity as a state and a process of being, acting like, and becoming a certain kind of person who is honest and trustworthy, consistently does the right thing and stands up for what is right despite the consequences. These behaviours are reflected in the Code, and a person with this integrity can be relied on to speak and act in a manner consistent with the right values, beliefs and principles (Webster and Baylis 2000).

The concept of trust underpins the entire NMC Code. Trust has been defined in the *Oxford Dictionaries* as the 'firm belief in the reliability, truth, or ability of someone or something'. People should be able to rely on your actions and decisions; they should be able to believe you and have confidence in you, your knowledge and your practice. People in your care should be able to trust you, as should your colleagues and the public in general.

Throughout your career, you may be faced with some moral uncertainty in situations in which you are unsure about what values or moral principles apply, or you are not entirely sure what the problem is (Jameton 1984). This can also occur when you may have some sense that something is wrong but you are not initially sure what it is or on what knowledge it is based (Webster and Baylis 2000). This has also been described as a 'gut feeling', and you may just need more information to explain and understand what you have observed (Hardingham 2004). It is what you do with these feelings and observations that is important.

Moral integrity means living up to your personal moral code so that you can sleep at night or live with yourself and carry on in the face of conflict (Laabs 2007). To do this, there is a need for coherence between your beliefs and behaviours (Webster and Baylis 2000). If you act in a way that is consistent with professional principles and commitments despite the consequences of doing so, you will be acting with integrity (Webster and Baylis 2000). McFall (1987) suggested that to demonstrate integrity you must stick to your principles despite any temptation you may face to do otherwise. To achieve this level of integrity, you will need to develop a critical perspective that will allow you to evaluate any social influences, and maintaining this integrity will require you to reflect on your principles and values and then justify them to others (Hardingham 2004). There must be a relationship between your values and your actions.

It is interesting to note that Ham (2004) found higher levels of integrity in senior baccalaureate students than in more experienced nurses, indicating that this high level of principled thinking diminished with years served as a nurse. Whilst a person with moral integrity may always try to do their best to do what is right, it may still not be easy; this difficulty may be compounded by time pressures, intimidation by others, lack of support in their beliefs, or ambiguous situations (Laabs 2011). Reflect on your own integrity when considering the practice scenario in Box 3.3.

Box 3.3

Practice scenario: integrity

You are in the final year of your studies, and your workload has increased. You, and some of your fellow students, are feeling pressurised by the deadlines you have to meet. One of your fellow students, Linda, has been approached by someone who will write an essay for her for a small fee. Linda tells you of her intention to submit this essay to the university as a summative assessment under her own name.

Questions

- Thinking about your professional code, what would your response be to this and why?
- Would this be classified as cheating?
- What action would you feel duty bound to take?

The public and your profession expect that you will act with integrity whilst in practice and in your personal life. According to your Code, Linda's actions would be classified as cheating, and if she cannot be trusted with following the correct procedures for academic work, how can she be trusted to practise in a professional manner, administer medication when required or accurately document care, for example. In addition, if you cannot be trusted and relied on to report Linda under these circumstances, how can you be relied on to report poor care or raise concerns about practice standards? This may sound extreme, but it all relates to the public and the profession's ability to trust you and your judgement.

Social media and technology

The use of information technology is unavoidable in nursing. It is used for recording patient data and communicating between professionals and agencies. Social media and e-mail are part of our everyday lives, and it may be easy to forget that any information transmitted by these means is not always as secure as we think it may be. Once information is posted on the Internet, it could potentially be accessed by people other than those for whom the initial communication was intended; it is not secure. Because we are so used to posting on the Internet, it is also easy to become complacent about what we write; often we communicate as though it were the same as having a verbal conversation with a friend. You may communicate something about your stressful day at work, and in describing your experience you may breach confidentiality or talk in an unfavourable or defamatory way about a colleague. Not only may this have an impact on your employment or on your registration if your employers or the NMC are made aware of it, but also you may be subjected to action under the Equality Act (2010). Under the Equality Act, bullying and harassment are unlawful; these behaviours make someone feel intimidated or offended, such as behaviour that includes spreading malicious rumours, unfair treatment, picking on someone, or regularly undermining someone. It is necessary therefore to be increasingly aware of how you use e-mail and social media, particularly as a registered nurse. You will not be able to use your private life as a defence.

Social media does have its place in the professional lives of nurses, and in fact the NMC (2011a) advocates the use of social networking and participates actively with the use of such media for communicating information and updates. The NMC nonetheless warns nurses and midwives that they could be risking their registration if they post comments about patients or colleagues because anything posted on a social networking site is in fact in the public domain. The NMC (2011a) produced tips to help you protect yourself when you are using social media (see Box 3.4). Now, consider the practice scenario in Box 3.5 and the questions posed.

Box 3.4

Summary of NMC tips for social networking (NMC 2011b)

1. **Be careful about privacy.** Once it is online, it is in the public domain, and your post can be copied.
2. **Know who your friends are.** Be aware of who your friends share your information with.
3. **Give your online life a health check.** Think about what your reasons are for using social networking sites.
4. **Watch your boundaries.** Maintain the boundaries between your personal and professional life.
5. **Think about confidentiality.** You must maintain confidentiality at all times in both what you say and photos you take.
6. **Do not put up with abuse.** Most sites will give you the ability to report abuse.
7. **Turn off your phone.** Think before you share.

The NMC provides information on the use of Facebook (http://www.nmc-uk.org/Get-involved/Events/NMC-staff-at-events/Facebook-trials-and-tribulations-social-networking-sites-and-their-joys-and-dangers/).

Box 3.5

Practice scenario: your personal life and social media

You belong to a group on Facebook that is a closed group that includes you and your student peer group. The idea of the group is to share experiences and learn from and support each other. You increasingly note, however, that posts from a small group of students on the site are becoming persistently derogatory. These posts range from derogatory comments about patients to negative comments about lecturers.

Questions

- Reflecting on the conditions that raise concerns about fitness to practice outlined in Table 3.2, what is your reaction to such behaviour?
- What is your responsibility as a student nurse to manage this behaviour?
- What, if anything, would you do about it?

Persistent inappropriate attitude or behaviour and unprofessional behaviour are classed as undesirable characteristics in a student nurse. In such a scenario, you have to question the values you hold about the profession and about the way in which you believe people should be cared for and respected. Can you trust this group of students, and can you be confident that this behaviour would not continue once they are qualified nurses? You could try raising these concerns with the wider group in the first instance, but you may need to follow this up with your lecturers. Would you want these students to be part of a profession that should be respected and trusted by the public?

Chapter summary

There are many expectations placed on you as a professional nurse, and this can feel like a heavy burden of responsibility, particularly when the media have a negative impact on the public image of nursing. The NHS, professional, statutory and public expectations are high, but fundamentally they are all linked and boil down to the fact that you should provide high standards of dignified and respectful care and behave in a way that is befitting a professional registered nurse. Throughout this chapter, you have had the opportunity to consider the relationship between public expectations of you as a nurse and quality and safety in nursing practice, to explore the media and public image of nursing and look at how you can promote a positive image of nursing, and to reflect on the possible public perceptions of your behaviour by looking at what constitutes fitness to practise. The way you conduct yourself in your professional and personal life and the way in which you demonstrate your knowledge, skill, performance and judgement have the potential to make the biggest impact on the image of nursing. Therefore, by meeting and exceeding the expectations discussed throughout this chapter you will have the biggest positive impact on the reputation of nursing and ultimately on standards of care.

References

Bridges, J.M. 1990. Literature review on the images of the nurse and nursing in the media. *Journal of Advanced Nursing* 15: 850–854.

Cabaniss, R. 2011. Educating nurses to impact change in nursing's image. *Teaching and Learning in Nursing* 6(3): 112–118.

Committee on Standards in Public Life. 2013. *Standards Matter. A Review of Best Practice in Promoting Good Behaviour in Public Life. Fourteenth Report of the Committee on Standards in Public Life.* London: HMSO. Available from: http://www.public-standards.gov.uk/wp-content/uploads/2013/01/Standards_Matter.pdf (accessed 10 December 2013).

Czarny, M.J., Faden, R.R., Nolan, M.T., Bodensiek, E., Sugarman, J. 2008. Medical and nursing students' television viewing habits: Potential implications for bioethics. *The American Journal of Bioethics* 8(12): 1–8.

Department of Health. 2013. *The NHS Constitution: The NHS Belongs to Us All.* London: Crown copyright. Available from: https://www.gov.uk/government/uploads/system/uploads/attachment_data/file/170656/NHS_Constitution.pdf (accessed 10 December 2013).

Department of Health. 2013. *The NHS Constitution for England.* Available from: https://www.gov.uk/government/publications/the-nhsconstitution-for-england (accessed 24 November 2013).

Equality Act. 2010. Available from: http://www.legislation.gov.uk/ukpga/2010/15/contents (accessed 17 October 2013).

Fletcher, K. 2007. Image: Changing how women nurses think about themselves. Literature review. *Journal of Advanced Nursing* 58(3): 207–215.

Francis, R. 2013. *Report of the Mid Staffordshire NHS Foundation Trust Public Inquiry. Executive Summary.* Available from: http://www.midstaffspublicinquiry.com/sites/default/files/report/Executive%20summary.pdf (accessed 19 December 2013).

Ham, K. 2004. Principled thinking: A comparison of nursing students and experienced nurses. *Journal of Continuing Education in Nursing* 35(2): 66–73.

Hardingham, L.B. 2004. Integrity and moral residue: Nurses as participants in a moral community. *Nursing Philosophy* 5: 127–134.

Henderson, V. 1978. The concept of nursing. *Journal of Advanced Nursing* 3: 113–130.

Jackson, D. 2009. Nursing on television: Are we being served? *Journal of Clinical Nursing* 18(16): 2249–2250.

Jameton, A. 1984. *Nursing Practice: The Ethical Issues.* Englewood Cliffs, NJ: Prentice Hall.

Keogh, B. 2013. *Review into the Quality of Care and Treatment Provided by 14 Hospital Trusts in England: Overview Report.* Available from: http://www.nhs.uk/NHSEngland/bruce-keogh-review/Documents/outcomes/keogh-review-final-report.pdf (accessed 19 December 2013).

Laabs, C. 2011. Perceptions of moral integrity: Contradictions in need of explanation. *Nursing Ethics* 18(3): 431–440.

Laabs, C.A. 2007. Primary care nurse practitioners' integrity when faced with moral conflict. *Nursing Ethics* 14(6): 795–809.

McFall, L. 1987. Integrity. *Ethics* 98: 5–20.

NHS England. 2013. *Putting Patients First: The NHS England Business Plan for 2013/14–2015/16.* Available from: http://www.england.nhs.uk/wp-content/uploads/2013/04/ppf-1314-1516.pdf (accessed 20 December 2013).

Nolan, M.P. 1995. *Standards in Public Life. First Report of the Committee on Standard in Public Life.* London: HMSO. Available from: http://37.128.129.237/wp-content/uploads/2012/11/1stInquiryReport.pdf (accessed 10 December 2013).

Nursing and Midwifery Council (NMC). 2008. *The Code: Standards of Conduct, Performance and Ethics for Nurses and Midwives.* London: NMC.

Nursing and Midwifery Council (NMC). 2010. *Standards for Pre-registration Nursing Education.* London: NMC.

Nursing and Midwifery Council (NMC). 2011a. *Facebook Trials and Tribulations: Social Networking Sites and Their Joys and Dangers.* Available from: http://www.nmc-uk.org/Documents/Events/Staff-at-events/Handout_Facebook-trials-and-tribulations-social-networking-sites-and-their-joys-and-dangers.PDF (accessed 10 December 2013).

Nursing and Midwifery Council (NMC). 2011b. *Guidance on Professional Conduct for Nursing and Midwifery Students.* Available from: http://www.nmc-uk.org/Documents/NMC-Publications/NMC-Guidance-on-professional-conduct.pdf (accessed 17 October 2013).

Nursing and Midwifery Council (NMC). 2012. *Summary of Patient Engagement Forum, 23 August 2012.* Available from: http://www.nmc-uk.org/patients-public/What-people-should-expect-from-a-nurse-or-midwife/Patient-Engagement-Forums/ (accessed 19 December 2013).

Oxford Dictionaries http://oxforddictionaries.com/definition/english/trust?q=trust) (accessed 26 April 2014)

Protection of Vulnerable Groups (Scotland) Act. 2007. http://www.legislation.gov.uk/asp/2007/14/contents (accessed 26 April 2014)

Radwin, L.E., Alster, K. 2002. Individualized nursing care: An empirically generated definition. *International Nursing Review* 49: 54–63.

Safeguarding Vulnerable Groups Act. 2006. http://www.legislation.gov.uk/ukpga/2006/47/contents (accessed 26 April 2014)

Smith, E.R., Mackie, D.M. 2007. *Social Psychology.* 3rd edn. New York: Psychology Press.

Suhonen, R., Papastavrou, E., Efstathiou, G., Tsangari, H., Jarosova, D., Leino-Kilpi, H., Patiraki, E., Karlou, C., Balogh, Z., Merkouris, A. 2012. Patient satisfaction as an outcome of individualised nursing care. *Scandinavian Journal of Caring Sciences* doi: 10.1111/j.1471-6712.2011.00943.x 372.380.

Summers, S., Summers, H.J. 2009. *Saving Lives; Why the Media's Portrayal of Nurses Puts Us All at Risks.* New York: Kaplan.

Ten Hoeve, Y., Jansen, G., Roodbol, P. 2013. The nursing profession: Public image, self-concept and professional identity. A discussion paper. *Journal of Advanced Nursing* doi: 10.1111/jan.12177.

The Safeguarding Vulnerable Groups (Northern Ireland) Order. 2007. http://www.legislation.gov.uk/nisi/2007/1351/contents/made (accessed 26 April 2014)

Weaver, R., Salamonson, Y., Koch, J., Jackson, D. 2013. Nursing on television: Student perceptions of television's role in public image, recruitment and education. *Journal of Advanced Nursing* 69(12): 2635–2643.

Webster, G., Baylis, F. 2000. Moral residue. In Rubin, S.B., and Zoloth, L. (eds.), *Margin of Error: The Ethics of Mistakes in the Practice of Medicine.* Hagerstown, MD: University Publishing Group, 217–232.

4 Nursing practice within ethical frameworks

Introduction

Ethics is closely linked to your personal and professional values and beliefs, and ethical principles can help you to deal with the dilemmas you will face. These dilemmas may involve the people in your care and other members of the healthcare team, but you may face dilemmas which exist because of differences between your personal and your professional values and beliefs. This chapter introduces you to concepts of ethical practice, which are key to ensuring that those in your care are treated with dignity and respect. A definition of ethics is offered, and some key ethical principles and theories are discussed. You are guided through some frameworks and models of ethics to help you with your decision-making, and the concept of advocacy is introduced.

Learning outcomes

By the end of this chapter, you will be able to

- Appreciate the range of ethical principles, frameworks and models and discuss their application to ethical decision-making in nursing practice;
- Recognise and address ethical challenges relating to people's choices and decision-making about their care;
- Reflect on your own virtues and personal versus professional beliefs.

What is ethics?

Over the last 30 years, nursing ethics has developed significantly, and whilst sharing the biomedical and philosophical principles of more traditional medical ethics, nursing ethics is now considered a respected discipline in its own right. Throughout your nursing career, you will observe and be involved in a range of decisions regarding the treatment of people in your care, from decisions regarding medical treatment; end-of-life decisions, including withdrawal of treatment and do not attempt resuscitation orders; and the allocation of resources, for example. However, you will be required to make a number of judgements and decisions yourself relating to the care you deliver on a day-to-day basis.

You will need to understand and be sensitive to the ethics behind the care you deliver and decisions you make, and ethical principles will help you to justify your practice. To be morally sensitive in practice, you will need to show the ability to recognise moral conflict and show an intuitive understanding of the person in your care in context, and you will need to show insight into the ethical consequences of decisions made (Lützén et al. 2000). Johnstone (2009) further suggested that the right action (an ethical action) is reliant on your ability to recognise moral issues, knowing how to take the ethical action, and your commitment and wish to achieve a moral outcome.

The word *ethics* is derived from the Greek word *ethos*, meaning 'character'. Ethics is the study of human conduct, principles and behaviour, more specifically moral behaviour. Ethics is a generic term to denote the number of different ways of examining and understanding moral life (Beauchamp and Childress 2013). Ethics is underpinned by what is 'good' or 'bad', and 'right' or 'wrong', moral decision-making and the circumstances behind these decisions. It also encompasses moral values, which are what guide individuals (see Chapter 1 for a more in-depth discussion of values). The word *moral* derives from the Latin *moralis*, meaning 'manner' or 'custom'. Ethics deals with questions about human morality and is central to decisions made in nursing and in health care in general. There are two main approaches to ethics that would be useful for you to consider for your nursing practice: non-normative ethics (virtues, personal and societal behaviour) and normative ethics (how people should live, what people should do, codes and norms, principles and theories). Tschudin (2003) suggested that nurses have primarily been concerned with normative ethics because of involvement in the wider aspects of health, whereas medicine has been more concerned with descriptive ethics, a type of non-normative ethics.

Whilst ethical theories provide frameworks or sets of morals to judge what is right or wrong in human conduct and good or bad in terms of human characteristics (Mappes and Degrazia 2001), it is for you to decide how, when and why these theories are applied.

Non-normative ethics

Two types of non-normative ethics exist, and both are non-normative because they aim to identify what 'is' rather than what 'ought to be'

(Beauchamp and Childress 2013). The first, descriptive ethics (the investigation of moral beliefs and conduct), relates to what you do, what and how you think and how you behave. It examines the moral choices and values held by a particular group or culture (Buka 2008). It does not question issues of right or wrong but does state what is so (Thompson 2008).

Secondly, meta-ethics (analysis of language, meaning of the terms *values*, *rights*, *obligation*, *morality*) discusses moral language. It looks to understand the nature of ethical properties and the meaning of the terms *virtue*, *obligation*, *duty*, *morality* and *rights*, for example. Meta-ethics is also used to question terms such as *right*, *wrong*, *good*, and *bad*.

Normative ethics

Normative ethics looks at the norms and principles used by people when they make moral choices or decisions, and it questions the duties or values underpinning moral choices (Thompson 2008). Normative ethics involves the application of codes, theories, rules, concepts and principles to your practice. It questions what you 'ought' to do in terms of your duty. People working with this field of ethics answer questions seeking to determine which norms that underpin guidance and conduct should be used and why (Beauchamp and Childress 2013).

Ethical principles and theories

Ethical principles are standards of conduct that constitute an ethical system (Johnstone 2009). They exist to guide you in the moral decisions you make in practice on a daily basis. The need to apply ethical principles is recognised internationally, but the way in which they are applied in different cultures can vary (Fry and Johnstone 2008). It is therefore important that you understand the cultural differences that may exist with people in your care.

Deontology

Deontology encompasses theories that are duty based and falls under the umbrella of normative ethics. In deontology, there are some actions that are in themselves wrong despite the consequences. Therefore, we would look at the nature of the action to judge the morality of the act. Gallagher and Hodge (2012) outlined the prescriptions within deontology as being 'to respect individuals for their own sake and not merely as a resource to help you achieve your own end or goals' (p. 4).

Immanuel Kant (1724–1804; a German philosopher) is well known for his theories of deontology also known as 'Kantian' ethics. Kant argued that to act in a morally right way, actions must be underpinned by obligation or duty, and that it is the motives of the person carrying out that act that are to be judged as right or wrong or as having moral worth. Hope et al. (2008) suggested that so duty-based theories can be used practically, these morally relevant duties must be specified. For example, if you reported poor standards of care because of your professional duty of care to a person who was being mistreated by a colleague, then this action would be judged as good or as having moral worth. However, if you carried out the same action through a duty to those in your care, but this time because you wanted to detract attention from the fact that you knowingly carried out poor care, your action would be judged as wrong and immoral because your motives were purely for your own gain. This example illustrates Kant's notion or test of the 'categorical imperative', which informs us of what 'should' be done regardless of self-gain. This categorical imperative is the standard of moral rules or principles (a maxim) from which all obligations and duties arise. The categorical imperative also tests the 'consistency of maxims'. For you, the Code (Nursing and Midwifery Council [NMC] 2008) is a maxim outlining the morally relevant duties for you as a nurse. Kant (1989) also added to the categorical imperative by saying that you must act to treat every person as an end and not only as a means.

Activity

Reflect on what you think your duties are in terms of your obligations as a professional.

Consequentialism

Consequentialism is a group of theories that look at the consequences of an action. The actions are right or wrong depending on the balance between the good and bad of the outcome. Here, an action is only morally right if it supports the best consequences or outcome. If, for example, you had to lie to a patient, it would be the consequences of that mistruth that would be morally relevant rather than the act of lying itself.

Utilitarianism is probably the most commonly known form of consequentialism. Jeremy Bentham (1748–1832; a British philosopher and social reformer) is regarded as the founder of modern utilitarianism, and John Stuart Mill (1806–1873; an English philosopher and civil servant) continued to expand on utilitarianism in his philosophy. The foundation of utilitarianism is the 'greatest-happiness' principle.

This purports that it is the greatest happiness, satisfaction or welfare of the greatest number that is the measure of right and wrong. This principle of 'utility' asserts that we should provide the maximum good over bad, or the least-possible bad if it is not possible to provide maximum good. Whilst Bentham and Mill discussed good in terms of happiness, much utilitarianism, particularly in relation to health care, is about the greatest health-related outcomes. However, regardless of the school of thought, all utilitarians use the principle of utility as the ultimate judgement of right and wrong.

When it comes to the allocation of health resources, this principle is important. If you only have a finite budget, under the utilitarian principle, you would spend that in a way that would benefit the most people in your care. This is in contrast to the deontological principle, by which, under the same circumstances and with the same budget, you could justify spending that whole budget on treating one person because you thought it morally right to give that person a fair chance to live, even if following the treatment that person died. Remember that with deontology it is the act itself that is judged rather than the outcome, whereas with utilitarianism it is the consequences of the act that are subjected to moral judgement. Now, draw on the content of this chapter so far to respond to the scenario in Box 4.1.

Box 4.1

Practice scenario: lying to a person in your care

You are caring for Mark, who is terminally ill. Mark's family and his doctors have decided not to tell him that he may die soon because they fear he will 'give up the will to live' if he knows about his prognosis. Mark is reluctant to take his medication, but you overhear the registered nurse saying to Mark that he should take his medication to help him get better.

Thinking back to the concepts of 'trust' and 'integrity' discussed in Chapter 2 and the ethical theories of consequentialism and deontology discussed in this chapter, consider whether the nurse's action to lie to Mark was morally right from both the consequentialist and the deontological perspectives. Justify your decision.

Rights theory

Rights are moral and legal principles of freedom or entitlement, including liberty and justice. Rights theory relates to rights that are determined in national or international ethical frameworks or laws that protect people from oppression, invasion of privacy and inequality and promote liberty, for example. The Human Rights Act (1998), discussed in more detail in Chapters 5 and 6, is an ideal example of such legal protection.

In rights theory, the moral action is an action that promotes and protects an individual's rights. Beauchamp and Childress (2013, p. 368) contended that a right 'positions one to determine by one's choices what others morally must or must not do'. Relating to your practice, this gives your patient (the possessor of the right) a justified claim to their rights (to consent to treatment, for example) and a justified claim against a healthcare worker or organisation should they breach those rights (Beauchamp and Childress 2013). You will therefore need to be familiar with what people in your care have the 'right' to receive in terms of health care and treatment.

Virtue ethics

Virtue ethics has a long history worldwide within moral philosophy and religious teaching (Banks and Gallagher 2009). It has grown in popularity over more recent years and particularly so in nursing and is therefore relevant to your nursing practice. It looks at the virtues that produce a good life (Thompson 2008). Buka (2008, p. 34) suggested that virtue ethics ask of any action 'What kind of person will I become if I do this?' or 'Is this action consistent with my acting at my best?' Buka (2008) further posited that virtues are the characteristics that enable us to act in ways that demonstrates the highest potential of our good character.

Plato, the classical Greek philosopher (ca. 427–347 BCE), recognised four cardinal virtues of prudence, temperance, courage and justice. Aristotle (384–322 BCE) followed by discussing the importance of being good, and the relationship between virtue and happiness (Banks and Gallagher 2009). Beauchamp and Childress (2013, p. 31) defined *virtue* as

> *a dispositional trait of character that is socially valuable and reliably present in a person, and a moral virtue is a dispositional trait of character that is morally valuable and reliably present.*

Scott (2003) concurred with this definition, adding that compassion and sensitivity are traits of character rather than duties of a role, and that there is a difference between someone with good intentions and the good or virtuous person. Beauchamp and Childress (2013) made distinctions between personal virtues and professional virtues in that professional virtues stem from role responsibilities, which are generally tied to employer expectations and professional standards. Beauchamp and Childress (2013, p. 33) highlighted six fundamental virtues necessary in nursing (and in medicine); a summary is provided in Table 4.1.

Table 4.1 Summary of Six Fundamental Virtues

Virtue	Summary of feature
Care	• Prominent in nursing ethics • Fundamental in relationships, practice, and action • Relates to 'caregiving', 'taking care of' and 'due care' • Relates to what nurses do and how they do it
Compassion	• There is active regard for another's welfare. • There is awareness of emotional response of sympathy, tenderness at another's suffering. • This is directed at others' pain, suffering, disability and sadness. • Nurses must understand feelings and experiences of those in their care and respond appropriately to show empathy (but empathy does not always lead to compassion). • The nurse who lacks compassion has a moral weakness.
Discernment	• This involves the ability to make the right judgement despite fears, external influences or personal attachments. • A person of discernment will understand and perceive what another person needs. • Discernment involves understanding how principles and rules apply in different circumstances.
Trustworthiness	• Trust is a confident belief and reliance on the moral character and competence of another person. • Being trustworthy is to merit confidence in your character and conduct. • Trustworthiness has the practical outcome of making health care effective.
Integrity	• Integrity is a primary virtue in health care. • It means soundness, reliability, wholeness, integration of moral character, objectivity, impartiality and fidelity in adhering to moral norms. • Integrity represents two aspects of your moral character: 1. A coherent integration of self-emotions, aspirations, and knowledge; 2. A trait of being faithful to moral values and standing up in their defence if necessary. • Professional integrity presents issues about wrongful conduct in professional practice.
Conscientiousness	• This trait links to conscience (mental faculty of and authority for moral decision-making). • You act conscientiously if you are motivated to do what is right and have tried hard to do what is right.

Source: Beauchamp, T.L., Childress, F. 2013. *Principles of Biomedical Ethics.* 7th edn. Oxford: Oxford University Press.

Banks and Gallagher (2009) have written extensively on virtue ethics and have related 'virtues' specifically to healthcare professionals. They discussed what is meant by 'character', a term used by Beauchamp and Childress (2013) in their definition of virtue explained previously, and concluded that character is different to personality in that it is associated with values and purpose. However, it would seem that it would be possible for a nurse to be of good character in the professional context but lack these moral exemplars in their personal life (Banks and Gallagher 2009). Banks and Gallagher (2009) do however, suggest that being of 'good' character in healthcare settings can depend on the organisation within which the individual works. This could explain why nurses who are normally viewed as of good character and demonstrate the virtues outlined in Table 4.1 have difficulty in reporting concerns, for example. Banks and Gallagher (2009) presented their list of virtues based on what they believed defines a well-rounded healthcare professional (see Table 4.2).

Activity

Thinking about virtues, reflect on what sort of person you would like to be, what sort of person you ought to be and how you should live your professional life. Write this down in a letter to yourself. Ask a friend or family member to post it to you in a year's time and then consider whether you have remained true to it, whether it was realistic, and whether you have developed further since you wrote this letter. Then, reflect generally on your character as a professional.

Principles of biomedical ethics

Beauchamp and Childress (2013) are widely known for their four ethical principles: respect for autonomy, non-maleficence, beneficence and justice. These principles underpin healthcare ethics in general and the care you deliver.

Respect for autonomy

Autonomy comes from the Greek words *autos*, meaning 'self', and *nomos*, meaning 'law', 'governance' or 'rule'. Autonomy is arguably the most important ethical principle underpinning the care you provide to people. Hope et al. (2008) suggested that this principle has had a significant impact on the demise of medical paternalism and has been central in the development of patient-centred care. In the healthcare setting, people in your care have the right to make decisions about their care. Autonomy is therefore the ability to make self-determining choices

Table 4.2 Summary of Banks and Gallagher's (2009) Virtues for Healthcare Professionals

Virtue	Summary of feature
Professional wisdom	• This wisdom requires you to understand the technical and professional artistry of your practice. • You need to be able to perceive the ethical dimensions of your practice. • You need to exercise moral imagination (particularly when it is difficult to care, be respectful or courageous). • You have to be capable of reflection and deliberation in your decision-making.

Care	• Care relates to these attributes:
	  • Attentiveness
	  • Responsibility
	  • Competence
	  • Responsiveness
	  • Integrity

Respectfulness	• This virtue involves the following:
	  • Self-regarding (self-respect)
	  • Other-regarding (respect for)
	  • The appropriateness of how you feel and act towards yourself and the appropriateness of your thoughts, feelings and actions towards others
	  • Valuing yourself and others
	  • Engaging with people

Trustworthiness	• It is expected that you will be relied on and behave accordingly. • You need to be aware that you are liable to be held responsible for your behaviour. • You should be able to give a credible performance as a responsible person.
Justice	• You need to be impartial. • You need to act fairly towards those to whom you owe an obligation. • You should act fairly in all situations in practice.
Courage	• You need to demonstrate the 'right' attitude towards fear and confidence. • Courage is needed to respond to everyday fears (e.g. the need to act on concerns about standards of care). • It is associated with resilience and resistance.
Integrity	• You need to demonstrate coherence of beliefs and ideals, consistency and reliability of action. • You need to show commitment to a set of professional values. • You need to be aware that values are interrelated. • You need the capacity to make sense of professional values. • You should be able to give a coherent account of beliefs and actions. • You should show the disposition to think, feel and act in accordance with core values. • You need a strength of purpose and the ability to implement these values.

and be self-governing (Johnstone 2009). To make an autonomous decision about their treatment, a person must not be 'controlled' by others (Newham and Hawley 2007), and this includes healthcare professionals. However, whilst the 'informed and competent' person has the right to refuse treatment, the respect for autonomy does not stretch to the right to demand any medical treatment or intervention that they want.

In their principle of autonomy, Beauchamp and Childress (2013, p. 101) defined the concept as

> *self-rule that is free from both controlling interference by others and limitations that prevent meaningful choice, such as inadequate understanding. The autonomous individual acts freely in accordance with a self-chosen plan.*

The authors focussed their theory of autonomy on 'autonomous choice' rather than on the capacity for governance and self-management. They suggested that even those who may be effective at self-management of their health could fail to make the right choices because of constraints caused by their condition, ignorance or coercion by others, for example. They further posited that if an individual places trust in a physician and gives consent to a procedure without fully understanding the information or without asking questions to inform their understanding, this is not an autonomous decision or authorisation of the procedure. This is particularly relevant to you as a nurse, as you need to promote the autonomy of those in your care. This is even the case where a person is detained in a mental health setting under the Mental Health Act (1983, as amended 2007) where they can still exercise their autonomy through, for example, meal choices (Beauchamp and Childress 2013).

In terms of 'choice', Beauchamp and Childress (2013, p. 104) presented three conditions of autonomous choosers: 'the premise that everyday choices of generally competent persons are autonomous':

1. **Intentionality**: Intentional action requires a person to act according to a plan (i.e. the act is not accidental). These intentional acts may not always be desired and not always what that person wants, but they are nonetheless intentional.

2. **Understanding**: If a person does not understand the action, then it is not autonomous. Understanding can be impaired because of illness, irrationality or immaturity. An autonomous action needs substantial but not complete understanding.

3. **Non-control**: A person must be free from control by external or internal influences. However, not all external influences are controlling.

The capacity for autonomous choice is discussed in Chapter 5. Beauchamp and Childress (2013) set out the following:

> *To respect autonomous agents is to acknowledge their right to hold views, to make choices, and to take actions based on their values and beliefs.*
>
> *(p. 106)*

Promoting autonomy involves a respectful attitude and behaviour, a disrespectful attitude or action is that which ignores, insults or demeans another person (Beauchamp and Childress 2013). Beauchamp and Childress (2013, p. 107) suggested the following moral rules to support the principle of respect for autonomy:

1. Tell the truth.
2. Respect the privacy of others.
3. Protect confidential information.
4. Obtain consent for interventions with patients.
5. When asked, help others to make important decisions.

Non-maleficence

Primum non nocere

'Above all [or first] do no harm' is enshrined in the Hippocratic requirement. Beauchamp and Childress (2013) stated that under this principle we are obligated to cause no harm to others, that is, 'one ought not to inflict evil or harm' (p. 152). Unfortunately, in any healthcare setting, people in our care are often subjected to harm by us when we administer injections, carry out painful procedures or administer harmful treatments (such as chemotherapy), for example, but this is overridden by the principle of beneficence, or doing good in the longer term (see the following discussion on beneficence). However, if people in our care are becoming malnourished or dehydrated because they are being neglected, then we are clearly causing them harm.

Beneficence

Although the principles of non-maleficence and beneficence can blur under certain circumstances, Beauchamp and Childress (2013) made clear distinctions between the two concepts. Whereas non-maleficence dictates that you should do no harm, beneficence requires you to actively take affirmative steps to help others and contribute to their welfare (Beauchamp and Childress 2013). They also identified two forms of beneficence: 'positive beneficence', which requires you to provide benefits to others, and 'utility', which requires you to balance benefits, risks and costs to produce the best overall results.

Your ability to always 'do good' for those in your care might be influenced by the resources available to you (Newham and Hawley 2007).

Justice

Justice in the healthcare context has parallels with justice in the wider context in that it is about society's expectation of what is right and fair. Beauchamp and Childress (2013) presented six theories of justice:

1. *Utilitarian* theory, focussing on maximising public utility (to each person according to rules and actions that maximise social utility)
2. *Libertarian* theory, emphasising individual rights to social and economic liberty (to each person a maximum of liberty and property resulting from the exercise of liberty rights)
3. *Communitarian* theory, derived from the concept of the good developed in moral communities (to each person according to the principles of fair distribution derived from conceptions of the good developed in moral communities)
4. *Egalitarian* theory, focussing on equal access to the goods in life (to each person an equal measure of liberty and equal access to the goods in life that every rational person values)
5. *Capability* theory, which identifies capabilities and forms of freedom deemed essential for a prosperous life (to each person the means necessary for the exercise of capabilities essential for a flourishing life)
6. *Well-being* theory, which emphasises essential core aspects of health and what is required to realise well-being (to each person the means necessary for the realisation of core dimensions of well-being)

Banks and Gallagher (2009, p. 170) suggested justice is about 'ensuring a fair allocation of harms and goods between people'. They further posited that this virtue of justice 'requires practical wisdom, and often courage in taking action' (p. 173). This principle of justice requires you to give 'due care' to all people regardless of race, gender, socioeconomic status or religion according to their nursing needs (Newham and Hawley 2007).

Using theories frameworks and models

Beauchamp and Childress (2013) provided eight conditions for the adequacy of an ethical theory and suggested that they should be judged on the applicability to a given situation. Box 4.2 summarises these conditions,

Box 4.2

Conditions for the adequacy of ethical theories (Beauchamp and Childress 2013, p. 352–354)

1. **Clarity**: An ethical theory should be as clear as possible.
2. **Coherence**: There should be no conceptual inconsistencies or contradictory statements in ethical theories.
3. **Comprehensiveness**: A theory should be as comprehensive as possible; that is, it can account for all justifiable norms and judgements.
4. **Simplicity**: A theory should have no more norms than are necessary; a few basic norms are preferable.
5. **Explanatory power**: A theory has sufficient explanatory power when it provides enough insight to help understand morality.
6. **Justificatory power**: The theory should provide grounds for justified belief.
7. **Output power**: The theory has output power if it produces judgements that were not in the original set of moral judgements on which the theory was constructed.
8. **Practicability**: The theory must be practical in its application; if it is unfeasible or can only be applied by a few people, then it is not practicable.

which may help you when considering which theory underpins moral decisions made in practice.

Schneider and Snell (2000) proposed a framework to approach ethical dilemmas; the framework encompasses a four-question model, called C.A.R.E. (considerations, actions, reasons, and experiences), which is based on tensions between you as the individual and the team. Whilst this was developed for use in medical education, they believed that it would transfer into healthcare settings in general. Abma and Widdershoven (2006) in fact evaluated it as effective for moral deliberation in mental health nursing practice. Table 4.3 summarises the four C.A.R.E. questions (Schneider and Snell 2000) and includes considerations for you.

Fairchild (2010) provided a model of nurses' ethical reasoning skills (NERS). This model was developed to help nurses review and make sense of ethical situations when faced with dilemmas and competing demands and values in healthcare environments (Fairchild 2010). Box 4.3 summarises the key aspects of this model.

Rest (1984) provided a useful four-component model of morality that may serve to help you in the development of your moral behaviour,

Table 4.3 C.A.R.E. Questions for Ethical Dilemmas

Questions	Individual or exterior?	Considerations for you
Question 1: What are my core beliefs, and how do they relate to this situation?	Individual: the intention of the individual	You need to understand your own core values and beliefs and recognise how these have an impact on the situation.
Question 2: How have I acted in the past when faced with similar situations? What do I like about what I have done? What do I not like?	Individual/exterior: reflects how the individual behaves and acts within a similar context	You need to question and reflect on the tensions between your values and your actual behaviour. For example, resources may prevent you from delivering the care that you believe to be right.
Question 3: What are the reasoned opinions of others about similar situations? What does our culture seem to say about this situation?	Collective: reflects outcomes of group processes and cultural codes	Here, your cultural code policies, procedures and the Code (NMC 2008) should be consulted to inform the situation.
Question 4: What has been the experience of others in the past when faced with similar situations? What do I like about what they have done? What do I not like?	Collective/exterior: concerns social behaviour within groups and society	You will need to understand how others have dealt with similar situations and what you can learn from that in light of your professional code.

Source: Schneider, G.W., Snell, L. 2000. C.A.R.E.: An approach for teaching ethics in medicine. *Social Science and Medicine* 51(10): 1563–1567.

Box 4.3

Model of nurses' ethical reasoning skills (Fairchild 2010)

- **Reflection:** critically reflective consciousness: being reflectively mindful of self and of individual or collective actions in the context of professional practice.
- **Reasoning:** dialectic reasoning: backward and forward thinking about a concept; taking in the big picture supports deeply reflective thought.
- **Review of competing values:** must be consciously managed on behalf of patients in a healthcare organisation as competing values can cause ethical and moral dissonance because they represent opposite or competing sets of assumptions.

which was viewed as the end product of four psychological processes: moral sensitivity, moral reasoning, moral motivation and moral character. These four components are dependent on each other; therefore, if you fall down in one of these areas, you will experience moral failure. These are summarised in Box 4.4.

Box 4.4

Four-component model of morality (Rest 1984)

1. **Moral sensitivity**: You will need to develop an awareness of how your actions affect other people and an awareness of different actions and the effect of these. It is about being sensitive to moral cues in a range of situations.
2. **Moral reasoning**: You will need to be able to judge which actions are right or wrong and morally justifiable.
3. **Moral motivation**: This is the importance you give to moral values and competing values in your moral judgements.
4. **Moral character**. This involves you developing courage. You may be morally sensitive and be motivated, but if under pressure you are distracted or discouraged, then you will fail morally.

Advocacy

Fry and Johnstone (2008) suggested that advocacy is one of the ethical concepts that underpin a nurse's decision making, and it is widely recognised within nursing codes of ethics as a 'professional ideal' and 'moral imperative' (p. 39). Put simply, advocacy has been defined as the 'means by which individuals can be empowered to express their opinion' (Gallagher et al. 2012, p. 71). Gallagher et al. (2012) suggested that advocacy could really empower patients who are, for a variety of reasons, unable to assert their needs.

Fry and Johnstone (2008) discussed three interpretations, or models, of nurse advocacy, the first being the 'rights patient protection' model, in which the nurse is seen to defend a patient's rights. There is then the 'values-based' decision model, by which the nurse helps the patient discuss his or her needs, interests and choices but without imposing the nurse's decisions or values on the patient. The third interpretation is the 'respect-for-persons' model, in which the nurse views the patient as a fellow human being entitled to respect. Here, the nurse protects the patient's dignity, privacy and choices.

Activity

- Consider which of these interpretations of advocacy fits with what you have observed in practice and why.
- Reflect on instances when you have seen advocacy practised well.

Personal versus professional beliefs

Throughout your life, your personal beliefs will have been informed by your upbringing, previous education, culture, religious and spiritual influences, and political beliefs. As a student, you will undergo a steep curve of professional socialisation, and this, to a greater or lesser extent, will continue as you progress through your career depending on your career path. Throughout this process, you will be exposed to a number of different cultures:

> *Culture consists of values and beliefs that a specific group hold in common ... a system of learned beliefs and customs that characterise the way of life for a particular society.*
>
> *(Settlemaier and Nigam 2007, p. 23)*

As a nurse, you will take on aspects of this culture: the shared beliefs of the culture of nursing as a profession.

Throughout your time as a student and on into your career as a registered nurse, you may encounter situations that will create some tensions between your personal beliefs and those required by your professional code. Box 4.5 presents an example of such a practice scenario that you could encounter; read it and reflect on your responses to this.

It is really important that you understand what you are feeling in circumstances such as those given in Box 4.5, and why, so that you can continue to practise with professional integrity.

Box 4.5

Practice scenario: personal versus professional beliefs

You are required to care for Arnold, who is currently serving a sentence at your local prison. Arnold requires help with his physical care as well as support for his depression and anxiety. He has a conviction for a sex offence, but you do not know the full details of this conviction.

Using the principles discussed in this chapter, reflect on your feelings about caring for Arnold. Are your personal beliefs likely to conflict with your professional duty of care? If they are conflicting, what could you do to resolve this conflict?

Chapter summary

Understanding ethical principles and the values underpinning these principles is key to your practice as a professional nurse. This chapter has taken you through a definition of ethics and introduced you to some of the frameworks and models that will help you to deal with a range of ethical dilemmas in your practice. You have had the opportunity to reflect on your duties and obligations as a professional nurse; use ethical principles to justify your decisions in relation to the morality of lying to a person in your care; reflect on what sort of person you would like to be, what sort of person you ought to be and how you should live your professional life; consider how you have observed advocacy in action; and reflect on a situation for which your personal beliefs may be incongruent with your professional beliefs.

References

Abma, T.A., Widdershoven, G.A.M. 2006. Moral deliberation in psychiatric nursing practice. *Nursing Ethics* 13(5): 546–557.

Banks, S., Gallagher, A. 2009. *Ethics in Professional Life. Virtues for Health and Social Care.* Basingstoke, UK: Palgrave Macmillan.

Beauchamp, T.L., Childress, F. 2013. *Principles of Biomedical Ethics.* 7th edn. Oxford: Oxford University Press.

Buka, P. 2008. *Patients' Rights, Law and Ethics for Nurses: A Practical Guide.* London: Hodder Arnold.

Fairchild, R.M. 2010. Practical ethical theory for nurses responding to complexity in care. *Nursing Ethics* 17(3): 353–362.

Fry, T.S., Johnstone, M.J. 2008. *Ethics in Nursing Practice. A Guide to Ethical Decision Making.* 3rd edn. Oxford, UK: Blackwell.

Gallagher, A., Hodge, S. (eds.). 2012. *Ethics, Law and Professional Issues. A Practice-Based Approach for Health Professionals.* Basingstoke, UK: Palgrave Macmillan.

Gallagher, A., Hodge, S., Pansari, N. 2012. Consent when capacity is compromised. In Gallagher, A., and Hodge, S. (eds.), *Ethics, Law and Professional Issues. A Practical-Based Approach for Health Professionals.* Basingstoke, UK: Palgrave Macmillan, 61–77.

Hawley, G. (ed.). 2007. *Ethics in Clinical Practice: An Interprofessional Approach.* Harlow, UK: Pearson Education.

Herring, J. 2013. *Medical Law.* 3rd edn. Harlow, UK: Pearson Education.

Hope, T., Savulescu, J., Hendrick, J. 2008. *Medical Ethics and Law: The Core Curriculum.* 2nd edn. Philadelphia: Elsevier.

Human Rights Act. 1998. Available from: http://www.legislation.gov.uk/ukpga/1998/42/introduction (accessed 17 October 2013).

Johnstone, M.J. 2009. *Bioethics: A Nursing Perspective.* 5th edn. Chatswood, Australia: Elsevier.

Kant, I. 1989. *Foundations of the Metaphysics of Morals.* 2nd edn. (Translated by Lewis White Beck.) London: Pearson. First published in 1785.

Lützén, K., Johansson, A., Nordström, G. 2000. Moral sensitivity: Some differences between nurses and physicians. *Nursing Ethics* 7(6), 520–530.

Mappes, T.A., Degrazia, D. 2001. *Biomedical Ethics.* 5th edn. Boston: McGraw Hill.

McAlpine, H., Krisjanson, L., Poroch, D. 1997. Development and testing of the ethical reasoning tool (ERT): An instrument to measure the ethical reasoning of nurses. *Journal of Advanced Nursing* 25: 1151–1161.

Newham, R.A., Hawley, G. 2007. The relationship of ethics to philosophy. In Hawley, G. (ed.), *Ethics in Clinical Practice: An Interprofessional Approach.* Harlow, UK: Pearson Education Limited, 76–100.

Nursing and Midwifery Council (NMC). 2008. *The Code: Standards of Conduct, Performance and Ethics for Nurses and Midwives.* London: NMC.

Rest, J.R. 1984. The major components of morality. In Kurtines, W.M., and Gerwitz, J.L. (eds.), *Morality, Moral Behavior, and Moral Development.* New York: Wiley, 24–38.

Schneider, G.W., Snell, L. 2000. CARE: An approach for teaching ethics in medicine. *Social Science and Medicine* 51(10): 1563–1567.

Scott, A. 2003. Virtue, nursing and the moral domain of practice. In Tschudin, V. (ed.), *Approaches to Ethics. Nursing beyond Boundaries.* Edinburgh: Butterworth Heinemann, 25–32.

Settlemaier, E., Nigam, M. 2007. Where did you get your values and beliefs? In Hawley, G. (ed.), *Ethics in Clinical Practice: An Interprofessional Approach.* Harlow, UK: Pearson Education, 15–34.

Thompson, M. 2008. *Ethical Theory.* 3rd edn. London: Hodder.

Tschudin, V. 2003. *Ethics in Nursing. The Caring Relationship.* 3rd edn. London: Butterworth Heinemann.

5

Nursing practice within legal frameworks

Introduction

The role of the nurse has changed substantially over recent years, particularly as nurses have taken on roles traditionally carried out by medical practitioners. This chapter introduces some of the key concepts associated with lawful practice. The different types of law are introduced to provide the context for nursing practice. The act of negligence is also explained, as is legislation that is particularly relevant for nursing care: the Mental Health Act (1983, amended 2007), the Human Rights Act (1998), the Mental Capacity Act (2005), the Children Act (2004), and the Equality Act (2010). Two further important legal principles underpinning your practice (consent and confidentiality) were discussed in Chapter 2 in relation to relevant legislation. Legislation related to safeguarding is discussed in Chapter 10.

Learning outcomes

By the end of this chapter, you will be able to

- Apply legal principles to act within the law when providing nursing care;
- Discuss legal capacity to make decisions about treatment and care;
- Apply statute law to the care you provide;
- Reflect on your own duty of care that is owed to people and recognise how negligence can arise.

Branches and types of law

The legal system is split into two types of law: criminal law and civil law. Criminal law is concerned with conduct that is damaging to social order (i.e. crime) and the legal punishment of such criminal offences. The Crown brings the case in criminal law against a defendant (the person who carried out the crime). In criminal law, to be successful, the case must be proven 'beyond reasonable doubt'; the defendant must be guilty of carrying out a criminal act, and malicious intent must be evident. You will see criminal law cases cited as *R* v. *Black*, with *R* representing Regina (the Crown) and the name *Black* as that of the defendant. Examples of crimes include theft, murder, assault or fraud. It is rare for charges to be brought against a nurse in a professional capacity under criminal law unless the nurse has engaged in a criminal act such as theft from a patient, murder, manslaughter or assault of a patient, for example. There are, however, high-profile cases of nurses who have been convicted under criminal law. For example, in 1993 Beverley Allitt was given 13 life sentences for murdering four children on the children's ward where she worked, attempting to murder another three, and causing grievous bodily harm with intent to a further six. In 2006, Benjamin Geen, 25, was found guilty of murdering 2 patients and causing grievous bodily harm to a further 15 patients. In 2008, Colin Norris was convicted and is currently serving a life sentence for the murder or attempted murder of five older women in his care.

Activity

Use a search engine to access reports about Beverley Allitt and Colin Norris and read about these cases.

- Reflect on how you feel about what these nurses did in terms of your values.
- How does their conduct contrast with the values of the nursing profession?

In relation to your nursing practice, you would see civil law dealing with actions in 'tort', which are civil wrongs. Here, a person's pre-existing legal right must have been breached, and disputes can occur between individuals, between individuals and organisations or between two organisations. A person in these instances brings action against another person or organisation because the person has suffered loss or personal harm. The person suffering the loss or harm would be known as the claimant, and the person or organisation against which the claim is made is known as the defendant. This type of dispute usually results in compensation being awarded to a 'victim' or claimant. You would see this type of case referred to using the names of the two parties involved, for example, *Black* v. *Baillie* or *Black* v. *Neverland NHS Foundation Trust*. The commonest form of tort that you may encounter is negligence, which may arise as a result of a breach of confidentiality or failure to gain consent. Negligence is discussed in greater detail in a separate section of this chapter.

In terms of your nursing practice, you will find law determined by statute, which means it is found in legislation (e.g. the Human Rights Act or the Equality Act) and is therefore set by Parliament. You will also find common law, also known as case law, having an impact on your practice. In this instance, a precedent has been set and the court's decision must reflect the decisions and principles of previous law if that exists. The previous case may not necessarily be health related, but the principles will still apply. You then have private law (law of tort, family law, welfare law, law of property and of contract) and public law (constitutional, criminal and administrative law), and these can both include statute and case law.

Statute law relevant to your practice

This section explores some legislation that is particularly relevant to your practice as a nurse: Human Rights Act (1998), Mental Capacity Act (2005), Children Act (2004), Mental Health Act (1983, amended in 2007), and Equality Act (2010). Chapter 2 explained the Data Protection Act of 1998 in relation to confidentiality.

The Human Rights Act (1998)

The Human Rights Act (1998) is a UK act of Parliament written to 'give further effect to rights and freedoms guaranteed under the European Convention on Human Rights' (http://www.legislation.gov.uk/ukpga/1998/42/introduction). The European Convention on Human Rights was amended in 2010 (Council of Europe 2010). The Human Rights Act incorporated the majority of the convention rights into UK law and came into force in 2000. It gives UK law the power to enact the rights detailed in the European Convention of Human Rights (a treaty that was signed in 1950 by the then-members of the Council of Europe, including the United Kingdom). Before the Human Rights Act, people in the United Kingdom who wanted remedy for a breach of their human rights would have to go to the European Court of Human Rights. The convention was signed to ensure that all member states act in accordance with a common standard of human protection. The convention protects around 800 million people in the 47 countries of the Council of Europe (Equality and Human Rights Commission [EHRC] 2012). These convention rights and rights included in the Human Rights Act are summarised in Table 5.1.

The Human Rights Act (1998) gives UK courts a solution for any breach of a convention right without involving the European courts. The act sets the requirements of public bodies within the United Kingdom to make sure that they adhere to the convention. The Human Rights Act enables us to challenge injustice and promote a society within which human rights are 'respected and enjoyed by all' (EHRC 2012, p. 5) and therefore

Table 5.1 Summary of Human Rights

The European Convention on Human Rights (1950)	The Human Rights Act 1998 Schedule 1 The Articles Part I
Article 2: Right to life	*Article 2*: Right to life
Article 3: Freedom from torture or inhuman or degrading treatment or punishment	*Article 3*: Prohibition of torture (including degrading treatment)
Article 4: Freedom from slavery or servitude or forced or compulsory labour	*Article 4*: Prohibition of slavery and forced labour
Article 5: Right to liberty and security	*Article 5*: Right to liberty and security
Article 6: Right to a fair trial	*Article 6*: Right to a fair trial
Article 7: Freedom from punishment without law	*Article 7*: No punishment without law
Article 8: Right to respect for private and family life, home and correspondence	*Article 8*: Right to respect for private and family life
Article 9: Freedom of thought, conscience and religion	*Article 9*: Freedom of thought, conscience and religion
Article 10: Freedom of expression	*Article 10*: Freedom of expression
Article 11: Freedom of peaceful assembly and association	*Article 11*: Freedom of assembly and association
Article 12: Right to marry	*Article 12*: Right to marry
Article 13: Right to an effective remedy	*Article 14*: Prohibition of discrimination
Article 14: Freedom from discrimination in the enjoyment of rights	*Article 16*: Restrictions on political activity of aliens
Article 17: Prohibition of abuse of rights	*Article 17*: Prohibition of abuse of rights
Article 18: Limitation on use of restrictions on rights	*Article 18*: Limitation on use of restrictions on rights

enables people to bring action against public authorities if they feel that their human rights have been breached.

Human rights affect us all on a daily basis, not just when under the care of a healthcare professional. These rights relate to the way in which our public authorities treat us, including National Health Service (NHS) organisations and the people working within those organisations. Human rights ensure that we can live without the fear of intrusion in our private lives, fear of degrading treatment, and fear of losing our life because of the acts or omissions of a public authority (EHRC 2012). In fact, in a poll, the EHRC (2012) found that 82% of people agreed that there should be a set of human rights standards for the way in which people are treated by public services (this would include the NHS). The Human Rights Act recognises that we should all be treated with dignity, respect and fairness. We should be protected under this act if we wish to voice our ideas or want to protest against something we feel to be unfair or something that threatens our liberty.

It is worth noting that there are three types of rights (EHRC 2012): absolute rights (these cannot be restricted or changed by the government), limited rights (for which the article identifies the circumstances when the government can lawfully restrict the right), and qualified rights (for which the government can lawfully restrict the rights in, for example, the interest of national and public safety and security, health protection, or to protect the freedom and rights of others in a democratic society) (EHRC 2012). Table 5.2 categorises convention rights under these three headings.

Table 5.2 Category of Rights

Category	Convention right
Absolute rights	• Right to life • Freedom from torture or inhuman or degrading treatment or punishment • Freedom from slavery or servitude or forced or compulsory labour
Limited rights	• Right to liberty and security • Right to a fair trial
Qualified rights	• Respect for private and family life, home and correspondence • Freedom of thought, conscience and religion, freedom of expression • Freedom of peaceful assembly and association • Freedom from discrimination

In relation to Article 2, the EHRC (2012) has been particularly critical of the care provided to people with mental health problems who are detained, the systems for investigating the death of a child in secure children's homes and the systems for investigating deaths of patients in mental health settings. Similarly, breaches of Article 3 have been highlighted by the EHRC (2012), which identified evidence of mistreatment of some users of health and social care services, concluding that people who use health and social care services might be at risk of inhumane or degrading treatment and that the state does sometimes fail in its duty to protect vulnerable people against ill treatment by others.

The Human Rights Act does have implications for your practice, and there are a number of examples of cases that have resulted in a breach of a person's rights while in care. For example, consider the case of *Savage* v. *South Essex Partnership NHS Foundation Trust* [2010] (see Box 5.1). In this case, Article 2 was breached by the staff working in that trust.

Box 5.1

Savage v. South Essex Partnership NHS Foundation Trust [2010]

Carol Savage was detained under the Mental Health Act at Runwell Hospital. At the hospital, she had been assessed as at risk of suicide. On July 5, 2004, she ran away and killed herself by walking in front of a train.

The judge found that the trust breached Article 2 because the staff had failed to do all that could have reasonably been done to avoid or prevent the suicide. Carol's daughter was awarded £10,000 in compensation.

The case of Winterbourne View (Department of Health [DH] 2012) is a shocking example of a breach of Article 3. In 2011, the BBC *Panorama* programme broadcast undercover film footage of staff at Winterbourne View Hospital (a private hospital in England) repeatedly assaulting and restraining the vulnerable people in their care. This included using cold showers as punishment, pulling their hair, forcing medication into their mouths and poking them in their eyes. As a result of the investigation into this appalling abuse, the hospital was closed, 11 of the staff pleaded guilty to the criminal offences of neglect or abuse, and 6 of the staff were sentenced to prison. These included Sookalingum Appoo, a registered nurse, jailed for 6 months for wilful neglect; Kelvin Fore, also a registered nurse, jailed for 6 months for wilful neglect; Wayne Rogers, jailed for 2 years for nine charges of ill treatment; Alison Dove (who suggested that the abuse arose because of boredom during her shift), jailed for 20 months for seven counts of abuse; Graham Doyle, jailed for 20 months for seven counts of abuse; Holly Draper, jailed for 12 months for two charges of abuse; and Daniel Brake, who was sentenced to 4 months imprisonment, suspended for 2 years, plus needed to perform 200 hours of unpaid work, for two counts of ill treating patients. It is interesting to note that the Mental Capacity Act (2005) (discussed separately in the following material) made the ill treatment or neglect of a person who lacks capacity (such as those in Winterbourne View) a criminal offence. Those found guilty of such a crime may be imprisoned for up to 5 years. Chapter 10, Box 10.2, gives an example of the application of this legislation to healthcare assistants who abused patients in a hospital ward.

It is really important that you are aware of the relevance of human rights to your care and make sure that this legislation is reflected when caring for people. An approach based on human rights involves putting human rights considerations at the centre of all policies and practices (Scottish Human Rights Commission [SHRC] 2009). This approach has been shown to foster a positive environment with reciprocal respect between patients and staff (SHRC 2009). Studies have shown that people agree on the importance of such values as fairness, freedom of expression, dignity and respect (EHRC 2012).

Activity

1. Visit the Council of Europe's website and look at the fact sheets relating to the European Convention on Human Rights (http://www.echr.coe.int/Pages/home.aspx?p=press/factsheets&c=).
2. Read *Human Rights: Human Lives. A Handbook for Public Authorities* by the Ministry of Justice (2006) (http://www.justice.gov.uk/downloads/human-rights/human-rights-handbook-for-public-authorities.pdf).

The Mental Capacity Act (2005)

The Mental Capacity Act (2005) applies to all health and social care workers providing health and social care and treatment in England and in Wales. It came into force in 2007 and is a legal framework to enable and safeguard people over the age of 16 who may be unable to make decisions because of mental health problems, dementia, a learning disability or head injury, for example. The act does not generally apply to people under the age of 16 years (see section on the Children Act of 2004 for the law relating to children). The act clarifies who can make decisions under such circumstances, including decisions about financial affairs and health treatment or care, lasting powers of attorney, and how these decisions should be made. It also provides guidance for assessing mental capacity to make decisions. The principles of the act are summarised in Box 5.2.

Box 5.2

Mental Capacity Act (2005) principles

1. A person must be assumed to have capacity unless it is established that he lacks capacity.
2. A person is not to be treated as unable to make a decision unless all practicable steps to help him to do so have been taken without success.
3. A person is not to be treated as unable to make a decision merely because he makes an unwise decision.
4. An act done, or decision made, under this Act for or on behalf of a person who lacks capacity must be done, or made, in his best interests.
5. Before the act is done, or the decision is made, regard must be given to whether the purpose for which it is needed can be as effectively achieved in a way that is less restrictive of the person's rights and freedom of action.

According to the Mental Capacity Act (2005), a person is able to make a decision if the person is able to

a. Understand the information relevant to the decision
b. Retain that information
c. Use or weigh that information as part of the process of making the decision
d. Communicate the decision (whether by talking, using sign language or any other means)

These criteria should be applied when assessing a person's capacity. The assessment of a person's capacity must be focussed on their ability to make the decision on something specific at the time it needs to be made, not on making a decision in general. An assessment should be carried out if there is any doubt regarding a person's ability to make a specific decision, and the outcome should be clearly recorded in notes about the person.

An example of this scenario is found in the case of *Re C (Adult: Refusal of Treatment)* [1994] (see Box 5.3). This is an interesting case because C was in fact unable to make everyday competent decisions because of his mental health. Yet, the court upheld his decision of refusal because he understood the information, was able to retain it, was able to weigh the information and make a decision, and could communicate his decision.

Box 5.3

Re C (Adult Refusal of Treatment) [1994]

C was a 68-year-old patient in Broadmoor Hospital. He had a history of chronic paranoid schizophrenia and expressed grandiose delusions (including having been an internationally renowned doctor). C developed gangrene in his leg, which a surgeon said required amputation. C refused this course of action and accepted that he might die as a consequence. Doctors argued that because of his delusions, C was unable to make a competent decision.

In all cases, every effort should be made to facilitate a person to make a decision. This includes providing all the information and any alternatives, communicating the information in a different way to make it easier to understand, considering the time of day when the decision is to be made, making the person feel at ease and offering additional support from a third party.

A person lacks capacity if

a. The person has an impairment or disturbance (e.g. a disability, condition or trauma or the effect of drugs or alcohol) that affects the way the mind or brain works, and

b. That impairment or disturbance means that the person is unable to make a specific decision at the time it needs to be made.

The inability to make a decision should not be confused with the inability to make the 'right' decision. Under the Mental Capacity Act, a person is entitled to make a decision that you may think is illogical or ill advised, but if they have the capacity to make that decision, then this should be respected. This may be frustrating for you, but in such circumstances it is important to reflect on why you feel this way and if it is because it conflicts with your values or beliefs (e.g. if a person refuses to have a blood transfusion for religious reasons even though this decision could be life threatening).

Activity

The Department for Constitutional Affairs (2007) published a code of practice that includes some useful scenarios relating to a person's capacity to make a decision. Visit the department's website to see if any of these scenarios are familiar and if they relate to the care that you deliver (http://webarchive.nationalarchives.gov.uk/+/http://www.dca.gov.uk/legal-policy/mental-capacity/mca-cp.pdf).

Best interests

The term *best interests* has been defined as follows:

> *A method for making decisions which aims to be more objective than that of substituted judgment. It requires the decision maker to think what the 'best course of action' is for the person. It should not be the personal views of the decision-maker. Instead it considers both the current and future interests of the person who lacks capacity, weighs them up and decides which course of action is, on balance, the best course of action for them.*
>
> *(British Psychological Society 2007, p. 7)*

A decision can be made in the best interests of a person in your care as long as the person lacks the capacity to make their own decision. A best interest decision should not be made based on a person's age or appearance or on unjustified assumptions relating to the person's behaviour or condition (Mental Capacity Act 2005). If it is necessary to make such a decision, the act details the criteria that the person making the determination should use (see Box 5.4).

Consider the case of *Re T (Adult: Refusal of Treatment)* [1992] discussed in Box 5.5. This case shows how a woman who was able to make a decision about her care had her decision overturned in her best interest as her health deteriorated. The Court of Appeal in this case decided that the doctors could disregard T's refusal of a blood transfusion primarily because of

Box 5.4

Criteria for establishing best interests (Mental Capacity Act 2005)*

The person making the best interest decision should consider the following:

- Whether it is likely that the person will at some time have capacity in relation to the matter in question and if it appears likely that the person will, when that is likely to be.
- Permit and encourage the person to participate, or to improve his or her ability to participate, as fully as possible in any act done for the person and any decision affecting the person.
- The person's past and present wishes and feelings (and, in particular, any relevant written statement made by the person when he or she had capacity).
- The beliefs and values that would be likely to influence the person's decision if the person had capacity.
- The other factors that the person would be likely to consider if able to do so.
- Consult anyone named by the person as someone to be consulted on the matter in question or on matters of that kind.
- Consult anyone engaged in caring for the person or interested in the person's welfare.
- Consult any deputy appointed for the person by the court regarding what would be in the person's best interests.

When the determination relates to life-sustaining treatment, the person making the decision must not, in considering whether the treatment is in the best interests of the person concerned, be motivated by a desire to bring about the death of the person concerned.

* (Department of Constitutional Affairs, 2005)

Box 5.5

Re T (Adult: Refusal of Treatment) [1992]

T, a 20-year-old woman, was pregnant when she was involved in a car accident. This resulted in premature labour and the need for a caesarean section. T's mother was a Jehovah's Witness, and shortly after a conversation with her mother, T signed a form refusing a blood transfusion even though she had not previously indicated any concerns about a transfusion. Following the stillbirth of her baby, T's condition deteriorated, and she was admitted to intensive care, where it was decided that she would die without a blood transfusion.

the undue influence exerted on her by her mother (see conditions for valid consent discussed in Chapter 2). This case also raised questions about fluctuating capacity. So, despite the fact that T was deemed to have the capacity to make decisions about her care at the time she made them, this changed as her condition deteriorated.

In terms of who can make a best interest decision, this all depends on the circumstances. This person may be referred to as the 'decision-maker', and the act includes the following examples:

- The carer most directly involved with the person at the time
- The doctor or other member of the healthcare staff responsible for carrying out the particular treatment or procedure
- If nursing or paid care is provided, the nurse or paid carer
- The attorney or deputy if a lasting power of attorney (or enduring power of attorney) has been made and registered

It is important that a person's best interests are reviewed regularly because their circumstances or ability to make a decision might change. This should be well documented in their case notes.

Deprivation of Liberty Safeguards and restraint

The Deprivation of Liberty Safeguards (DOLS) involve an amendment to the Mental Capacity Act and came into force in 2009, following a European Court of Human Rights ruling. DOLS apply to people in hospitals and care homes registered under the Care Standards Act of 2000, whether receiving the care through private arrangements or through public funding (DH 2009). The DOLS provide legal protection for people in England and Wales who are over 18 years old and lack the capacity to consent to arrangements for their care and treatment. DOLS are discussed in more detail with application to practice in Chapter 10 in relation to safeguarding. Chapter 10 also includes discussion of safeguards relating to use of restraint in nursing practice, with reference to the Mental Capacity Act.

The Children Act of 2004

In 2003, a Green Paper, *Every Child Matters,* was published by the UK government proposing policy and legislative changes to maximise opportunities and minimise risks for children and young people in England. These changes focussed on managing services more effectively concerning the needs of children, young people and their families. The Green Paper outlined clear accountability for children's services to ensure more collaborative working between health and social care professionals and a greater focus on safeguarding children.

Following a consultation on the Green Paper and in response to the *Victoria Climbié Inquiry* (Laming 2003), the Children Act was published in 2004.

The Children Act (2004) defines a child as a person up to the age of 18 and a person aged 18, 19 or 20 years who

a. Has been looked after by a local authority at any time after attaining the age of 16; or

b. Has a learning disability.

However, other definitions of a *child* do exist. For example, the United Nations Convention on the Rights of the Child stated that a child refers to any person below the age of 18 years unless, under the law applicable to the child, majority is attained earlier (Convention on the Rights of the Child 1989). The Department for Constitutional Affairs (2007) offered a further definition in which children are seen as people under the age of 16 and young people as those who are between the ages of 16 and 17. It may be worth using the definition offered by the Children Act as a starting point.

The Children Act advocates a child-centred approach to the provision of care and social services. This child-centred approach includes identifying any needs early to ensure an intervention is in place before the need escalates. Whilst you may not feel you have much influence over the running of a service at this stage in your career, you can still play a big part in making sure you adopt a child-centred approach and that you involve all necessary agencies in the care you deliver.

You can also directly influence care by making sure you have regard to the importance of parents and other persons caring for children in improving the well-being of children (Children Act 2004) and strive to improve the well-being of children in your care by

a. Improving their physical and mental health and emotional well-being

b. Protecting them from harm and neglect

c. Facilitating education, training and recreation

d. Promoting the contribution made by them to society

e. Improving their social and economic well-being (Children Act 2004)

Consider the scenario in Box 5.6, with reference to the Children Act, and reflect on the questions posed.

Box 5.6

Practice scenario: improving the well-being of children

Alice is 11 years old and is the main carer for her mother, Patricia, who has multiple sclerosis. You are visiting Patricia as a member of the multi-disciplinary team involved in her care. Alice is often late for school, particularly when Patricia is having a 'bad day' as Alice puts it. Alice also often misses afterschool activities because she has to rush home to Patricia. Recently, Alice started at a different secondary school to most of her friends, and she is finding it difficult to make new friends.

In your role, how could you

a. Help to improve Alice's physical and mental health and emotional well-being?
b. Protect Alice from harm and neglect?
c. Facilitate Alice's education, training and recreation?
d. Promote the contribution Alice can make to society?
e. Improve Alice's social and economic well-being?

The Mental Health Act of 1983 (amended in 2007)

Mental health is the concern of every practitioner, and you will care for children and adults with mental health needs and disorders in varied care settings. The Mental Health Act (2007) is an act that amends the Mental Health Act of 1983; the Domestic Violence, Crime and Victims Act (2004); and the Mental Capacity Act (2005) in relation to mentally disordered persons. It is necessary to review the 1983 and 2007 acts in conjunction with each other. The definition of mental disorder was reclassified in the 2007 act, replacing the four categories of 'mental illness', 'arrested or incomplete development of mind', 'psychopathic disorder' and 'any other disability or disorder of mind', with 'any disorder or disability of the mind'. People with learning disabilities will not be considered to be suffering from a 'mental disorder' unless the disability is 'associated with abnormally aggressive or seriously irresponsible conduct'. Dependence on drugs or alcohol is no longer categorised as a mental disorder.

The Mental Health Act (1983) focussed on strengthening patients' rights to seek independent reviews of their treatment, whereas the 2007 Mental Health Act focusses more on public protection and risk management. It also makes patient compliance with treatment a statutory requirement by extending the powers of compulsion and introducing compulsory community treatment orders. Community treatment orders replace the 'supervised discharge' of the 1983 act. If certain criteria are met, patients who are discharged from the hospital will be allowed to live at home under supervision to ensure they continue with the medical treatment that they need. Under Section 17E, responsible clinicians can recall patients to the hospital if the patients do not comply with conditions such as making him- or herself available for examination.

Adults requiring inpatient treatment can be informally admitted of their own accord or detained under Sections 2, 3 and 4 of the Mental Health Act.

Section 2 of the Mental Health Act relates to admission for assessment. An approved mental health professional or nearest relative can apply for admission for assessment, which can last up to 28 days, but either party must have seen the person in the previous 14 days. The admission must be authorised by two doctors, who should both agree that

a. The patient is suffering from a mental disorder of a nature or degree that warrants detention in a hospital for assessment; and

b. The patient ought to be detained for his or her own health or safety or the protection of others.

The patient can be discharged by a responsible clinician, hospital manager, the nearest relative, or the mental health review tribunal, which can determine whether patients should be formally discharged or detained in hospital.

Section 3 of the Mental Health Act relates to admission for treatment. Here, a nearest relative can apply for admission or, if the nearest relative does not object, has been displaced, or it is not reasonably practicable to consult him or her, an approved mental health professional can do the same. Detention can last for up to 6 months after two doctors have confirmed that

a. The patient is suffering from a mental disorder of a nature or degree that makes it appropriate for the patient to receive medical treatment in a hospital;

b. The treatment is in the interest of his or her health and safety and the protection of others; and

c. Appropriate treatment must be available for the patient.

Admissions under Section 3 can be renewed for a further 6 months and thereafter for periods of 12 months at a time. The patient can be discharged by the responsible clinician, hospital manager, nearest relative (if the responsible clinician refuses, the nearest relative can apply to a mental health review tribunal within 28 days) or mental health review tribunal.

Section 4 of the Mental Health Act relates to admission for assessment in an emergency. In this case, an approved mental health professional or nearest relative can apply for admission, having seen the patient in the previous 24 hours. A patient can be detained for up to 72 hours after one doctor has confirmed that

a. The detention is of 'urgent necessity'; and

b. Waiting for a second doctor to approve the detention under Section 2 would cause an 'undesirable delay'.

In all cases, hospital managers must ensure that patients aged under 18 admitted to the hospital for a mental disorder are accommodated in an environment that is 'age appropriate' (i.e. suitable for their age).

Section 136 details police powers to remove a person deemed to be mentally disordered and requiring immediate care and control to a place of safety, which may include a hospital or care home; a police station should be considered only as a last resort. People can be held under Section 136 for up to 72 hours, within which time they should be assessed by a doctor and an approved mental health professional.

If a person is detained long term under the Mental Health Act, the 'appropriate treatment test' (previously the 'treatability test') should be applied. This means that professionals must guarantee the availability of case-appropriate medical treatment (including psychological intervention) for the detention to be valid.

In terms of the professional roles, the 'approved mental health practitioner' (previously the 'approved social worker') role can be filled by anyone with experience in supporting people with mental health problems, such as nurses, occupational therapists and psychologists. Responsible medical officers no longer have to be medical practitioners; this role is now taken by the 'responsible clinician' role, which could be filled by social workers or any of the other professions listed previously. However, recommendations for detentions under Sections 2 and 3 of the act will still have to be made by two 'registered medical practitioners'.

The Equality Act (2010)

The Equality Act (2010) replaced previous anti-discrimination laws (Equal Pay Act of 1970, Sex Discrimination Act of 1975, Race Relations Act of 1976, Disability Discrimination Act of 1995) with a single act, making the law easier to understand. It legally protects people from discrimination in the workplace and in wider society and establishes protected characteristics (detailed in Section 4 of the act) that cannot be used to treat people unfairly. It sets out the different ways in which it is unlawful to treat someone. It is against the law to discriminate against people at work, in education, as a consumer, when using public services, when buying or renting property or as a member or guest of a private club or association because of

1. **Age**: an individual person or an age group
2. **Disability**: a person with a physical or mental impairment and the impairment has a substantial and long-term adverse effect on their ability to carry out normal day-to-day activities
3. **Gender reassignment:** if the person is proposing to undergo, is undergoing or has undergone a process (or part of a process) for the purpose of reassigning the person's sex by changing physiological or other attributes of sex
4. **Marriage and civil partnership**: if the person is married or a civil partner
5. **Pregnancy and maternity**
6. **Race**: colour, nationality, ethnic or national origin, a person of a particular racial group
7. **Religion or belief**: any religion or lack of religion; belief means any religious or philosophical belief or lack of belief
8. **Sex:** a man or a woman
9. **Sexual orientation:** a person's sexual orientation towards someone of the same sex, opposite sex or either sex.

A variety of different forms of discrimination exists:

- **Direct discrimination**: treating someone with a protected characteristic less favourably;
- **Indirect discrimination**: putting rules in place that apply to everyone but doing so puts people with a protected characteristic at an unfair disadvantage;
- **Harassment**: unwanted conduct relating to a protected characteristic that violates someone's dignity or creates an intimidating, hostile, degrading, humiliating or offensive environment;
- **Victimisation:** treating someone unfairly because they have complained about discrimination or harassment, giving false information or making false allegation against someone, or an allegation made in bad faith, failure to make reasonable adjustments to accommodate a person's disability.

As a result of the Equality Act, your employers have a clear duty not to discriminate. Your employer

- Must not discriminate in deciding to whom to offer employment
- Must not discriminate in offering opportunities for promotion, access to training or other benefits
- Must not victimise a person
- Has a duty to make reasonable adjustment for an employee with a disability
- Must not harass a person

It is important that you promote a culture that values equality and diversity. This relates to your colleagues as well as those in your care. This can be difficult, and sometimes you might not realise that there is discriminatory practice occurring around you because it might be subtle. It is important to think about how these subtle practices might affect people so you can improve the lives of colleagues and people in your care.

Activity

Reflecting on your values, write three pledges that outline the ways in which you can strive to foster a culture that promotes equality.

Negligence

Medical malpractice has been defined as 'any unjustified act or failure to act upon the part of a doctor or other healthcare worker which results in harm to the patient' (Stauch et al. 2002, p. 295). Negligence falls under the auspices of tort law. If someone in your care suffers harm because of professional negligence, that person will be entitled to claim compensation. However, it is unusual for nurses to be sued individually; it is more likely that the claimant will bring action against your organisation as the organisation is vicariously liable. Regardless of who the action is brought against, to succeed in their claim for compensation for negligence, a claimant must be able to prove duty, breach, causation and damage as follows:

1. That a duty of care existed, that is, the defendant owed the claimant a legal duty of care

2. That the defendant breached that duty of care

3. That the claimant suffered harm or injury as a direct result of the breach of the duty of care

Beauchamp and Childress (2013) suggested that negligence is the absence of due care and the departure from your professional standards that determine due care; they identified two types of situations under which negligence occurs:

> 1. *Advertent negligence or recklessness—intentionally imposing unreasonable risks of harm (if you knowingly fail to carry out a procedure for example)*
> 2. *Inadvertent negligence—unintentionally but carelessly imposing risk of harm (for example if you unknowingly did something harmful but you should have known not to).*
>
> *(p. 155)*

The term *duty of care* has a moral effect and is based on our obligations to others with whom we have a relationship (Buka 2008). In health care (including nursing), it is generally easy to establish that a duty of care exists. Once a person enters into your care, you have a duty of care to them, and the law imposes this duty of care: 'A legal duty of care is to any person whom we ought reasonably to foresee might be affected by our act or omission' (Gallagher and Hodge 2012, p. 12), that is, anyone who, as a nurse, you may foreseeably harm (Herring 2013). Beauchamp and Childress (2013) discussed the notion of 'due care', which they said is underpinned by the principle of non-maleficence:

> *Due care is taking appropriate care to avoid causing harm, as the circumstances demand of a reasonable and prudent person.*
>
> *(p. 154)*

The law did not recognise a general principle in tort apportioning liability for carelessness until the 1930s with the case of *Donoghue* v. *Stevenson* (Deakin et al. 2012). This case established the principle of duty of care (see Box 5.7). Whilst this was not a healthcare-related case, it still stands in claims of negligence in healthcare malpractice. In *Donoghue* v. *Stevenson* [1932], Lord Aitkin established the 'neighbour principle', by which he stated that you must not injure your neighbour, with your neighbour being someone who is closely and directly affected by your acts or omissions.

Box 5.7

Donoghue v. *Stevenson* [1932]

The claimant, Mrs Donoghue, went to a café with a friend who purchased a bottle of ginger beer for her. Mrs Donoghue drank half of the ginger beer before pouring the rest into a glass. Mrs Donoghue then found the remains of a decomposed snail in the rest of the ginger beer. Mrs Donoghue claimed that she suffered illness as a result of drinking this tainted ginger beer. The judges concluded that manufactured goods should reach the consumer in the state intended. Therefore, the manufacturer owed the consumer a duty of care to ensure the purity of the product. Mrs Donoghue was therefore awarded damages because the manufacturer had failed in its duty of care to ensure that the goods would not harm her.

The test for duty of care was established by Lord Bridge in *Caparo Industries plc* v. *Dickman* [1990], and this test may be applied to establish duty of care:

1. Foreseeability of damage arising from the act or omission exists.
2. There is a sufficient relationship of proximity between the parties.
3. As a matter of legal policy, it is fair, just and reasonable that a duty of care should exist.

Once a duty of care has been established, the second aspect of negligence that must be proven is that the existing duty of care has in fact been breached. By accepting responsibility for those in your care, you must ensure that any necessary procedures or care tasks are carried out competently. If not, you will have breached your duty of care because the law of negligence only requires you to exercise reasonable care in the performance of your nursing skills (McHale and Fox 2006).

The case of *Bolam* v. *Friern Hospital Management Committee* [1957] (see Box 5.8) became the test case from which the principle called the 'Bolam test' developed and is applied. According to this case, duty of care will have been breached if the person carrying out that breach acted in a way that a reasonable person in the same circumstances would not act. At the time of this case, three different practices were in use: manual restraint of the chin only, rigid restraint and muscle relaxants. Although it may now be accepted practice to administer muscle relaxants, in the 1950s electroconvulsive therapy (medically induced seizures) was a relatively new psychiatric procedure. However, the principle from this case remains. This principle is essentially that of the reasonable body of evidence; that is, if a doctor or a nurse acts in a way that is supported by a reasonable body of evidence, the doctor or nurse has not been negligent. In claims of negligence, this principle resulted in the Bolam test, which considers whether the healthcare professional falls below the standard of the skilled professional exercising and professing to have that skill. For example, if you are a newly qualified nurse, you admit to being competent in a particular skill, and you carry out that skill incorrectly,

Box 5.8

Bolam v. Friern Hospital Management Committee [1957]

John Bolam was a psychiatric patient suffering from a mental illness that resulted in him experiencing depression. He was advised by a consultant at Friern Hospital to undergo electroconvulsive therapy. He signed a consent form, but he was not informed of the injuries that can occur as a result of the convulsions that the procedure can cause. He received the treatment and experienced these convulsions, which resulted in fractures to his pelvis and dislocation of his hips. Bolam successfully claimed damages against Friern Hospital, alleging negligence because he was not given muscle relaxants prior to the procedure.

you may be judged against the standard expected of newly qualified nurses and what they would do under the same circumstances. However, it is not sufficient to cite inexperience as a reason for incompetence.

In 1997, another case resulted in the adoption of a more robust version of the Bolam test (Jackson 2010). The case of *Bolitho* v. *City and Hackney Health Authority* [1998] (see Box 5.9) established that the views of experts must be defensible and be capable of withstanding 'logical analysis'. The registrar in the *Bolitho* case said that she would not have intubated Patrick if she had attended him, even though it may have saved him, because of the risks. Opposing sides argued the case, presenting different evidence to support their views. Although the court found that the registrar was not negligent in her actions and had not breached her duty of care, an important legal principle arose from this case. Lord Browne-Wilkinson established that the court must be satisfied that expert opinion relied on can demonstrate such an opinion on a reliable basis and that opinion must be justified and there must be 'reason' for the opinion. This reinforces the need to keep up to date with best practice and evidence (see Chapter 12 for more on the importance of evidence-based practice).

Box 5.9

Bolitho v. *City and Hackney Health Authority* [1998]

Two-year-old Patrick Bolitho was admitted to the hospital with breathing difficulties following an episode of croup. His breathing appeared to be temporarily obstructed; therefore, the nurse called for the senior paediatric registrar. Neither the registrar nor the senior house officer responded. Patrick's condition deteriorated, and he subsequently suffered a cardiac arrest, which resulted in brain damage and then his death.

There must be damage or harm caused following the breach to make a successful claim in negligence. There is likely to be some identified harm or injury; otherwise, the claimant would not proceed far with the claim. The burden of proof is on the claimant to prove that loss or injury. However, proving that the damage was caused by the breach is often the difficult part of the process. As highlighted, having established that the person receiving the care has been damaged or injured in some way, it is necessary to establish whether the damage was caused as a direct result of that breach. The claimant must be able to prove that the harm resulted from the breach, based on the balance of probabilities. The claimant must also be able to prove the proximity in the relationship, as in *Caparo Industries plc* v. *Dickman* [1990].

The question to ask here is what would have happened but for the defendants' negligence (Brazier and Miola 2000). Would the injury or harm have occurred despite the act or omission by the defendant? This is known as the 'but for' test or principle. Remember that this negligence relates to acts (doing something that causes harm) or omissions (failing to do something, which then resulted in harm). This principle is illustrated in the case of *Barnett* v. *Chelsea & Kensington Hospital Management Committee* [1968] (see Box 5.10). The judge said that even if the patient had been admitted, he would have died anyway because the antidote was not readily available and it could not have been administered in time. The conclusion of the case was that the hospital owed the deceased a duty of care because of proximity; the duty of care was breached (because it was reasonable that these men were examined at the request of the nurse) and the care therefore fell below the required standard. However the failure to examine did not cause the death and therefore the judge ruled that, while the hospital (and the doctor) had been negligent, the hospital could not be held liable for the death because the patient would have died anyway. Causation could not be proven.

Box 5.10

Barnett v. *Chelsea & Kensington Hospital Management Committee* [1968]

While on duty, three night watchmen drank tea, but soon after drinking the tea all three became unwell and started vomiting. They attended their local accident and emergency department at about 8 a.m., where they were seen by a nurse. The nurse phoned the doctor, who did not go and see the patients, but instead told the nurse to discharge the men home to go and see their own general practitioners. One of the men died about 4 hours later. The postmortem showed that the death was caused by arsenic poisoning, which was rare. For arsenic poisoning, the antidote was not readily available and needed to be administered as soon as possible after the poisoning. The deceased's widow brought a claim of negligence against the hospital.

Now, read the scenario in Box 5.11 and consider the questions asked.

Box 5.11

Practice scenario: duty of care and negligence

Florence is 74 years old and has dementia. She has been admitted to hospital with dehydration. She has been in hospital for 8 hours but has not received any fluids, and there has been no assessment of her fluid balance needs. Florence dies a day later, and there is an inquest into her death.

Questions

In relation to the role of the nurse, apply the principles of duty, breach, damage and causation in answering the following questions:

1. Do the nurses owe a duty of care to Florence?
2. Was the duty breached and why?
3. Is there a link between the death and the breach?
4. Is there a case of negligence to answer? If so, why?

In relation to the practice scenario in Box 5.11, you could argue the following points:

- The nurse owed a duty of care to Florence because of the proximity principle and because of professional requirements.
- The duty of care was breached because the care fell below the required standard.
- If Florence's death can be linked directly to her dehydration, then causation can be proven on the grounds that the omission by the nurse to ensure she was appropriately rehydrated directly resulted in her death.
- There would be a case to answer because breach of duty and causation can be proven.

Chapter 10 focusses on safeguarding, which is also relevant to situations like Florence's, particularly in terms of neglect.

Chapter summary

This chapter introduced you to some of the key legal principles underpinning the care delivered on a daily basis and to legislation that is particularly relevant to nursing practice. You have had the opportunity to consider the importance of law in care delivery and link this to your duty of care and your practice. Understanding the legal principles that underpin care delivery is essential for ensuring that those in your care receive the service to which they are legally entitled. Practising in a way that is underpinned by these legal principles will also help to protect you should there be any question of negligence. After the introduction provided by this chapter, you can read further into the legal dimensions of nursing; there are a number of textbooks that focus on nursing and health care within a legal context. Also, be aware that legislation is continually evolving and amended, so you will need to ensure that you remain up to date with legal aspects of nursing throughout your career.

References

Barnett v. *Chelsea & Kensington Hospital Management Committee* [1968]. 1 All ER 1068.

Beauchamp, T.L., Childress, F. 2013. *Principles of Biomedical Ethics.* 7th edn. Oxford: Oxford University Press.

Bolam v. *Friern Hospital Management Committee* [1957]. 1 WLR 582.

Bolitho v. *City and Hackney Health Authority* [1998]. AC 232.

Brazier, M., Miola, J. 2000. Bye-bye Bolam: A medical litigation revolution? *Medical Law Review* 8: 85–114.

British Psychological Society. 2007. *Best Interests: Guidance on Determining the Best Interests of Adults Who Lack the Capacity to Make a Decision (or Decisions) for Themselves* [England and Wales] British. Leicester, UK: Psychological Society.

Buka, P. 2008. *Patients' Rights, Law and Ethics for Nurses: A Practical Guide.* London: Hodder Arnold.

Caparo Industries plc v. *Dickman* [1990]. 2 AC 605.

Care Standards Act. 2000. http://www.legislation.gov.uk/ukpga/2000/14/contents (accessed 26 April 2014).

Children Act. 2004. Available from: http://www.legislation.gov.uk/ukpga/2004/31/contents (accessed 17 October 2013).

Convention on the Rights of the Child. 1989. Available from: http://www.ohchr.org/Documents/ProfessionalInterest/crc.pdf (accessed 1 September 2013).

Council of Europe. 2010. *European Convention of Human Rights.* Available from: http://www.echr.coe.int/Documents/Convention_ENG.pdf (accessed 17 October 2013).

Data Protection Act. 1998. http://www.legislation.gov.uk/ukpga/1998/29/contents (accessed 26 April 2014).

Deakin, S., Johnston, A., Markesinis, B. 2012. *Tort Law.* 7th edn. Oxford: Oxford University Press.

Department for Constitutional Affairs. 2005. *Mental Capacity Act. 2005, Summary.* Available from: http://webarchive.nationalarchives.gov.uk/+/http://www.dca.gov.uk/menincap/legis.htm (accessed 17 October 2013).

Department for Constitutional Affairs. 2007. *Mental Capacity Act. 2005 Code of Practice.* Available from: http://webarchive.nationalarchives.gov.uk/+/http://www.dca.gov.uk/legal-policy/mental-capacity/mca-cp.pdf (accessed 17 October 2013).

Department of Health (DH). 2009. *Reference Guide to Consent for Examination or Treatment.* 2nd edn. London: Department of Health. Available from: https://www.gov.uk/government/publications/reference-guide-to-consent-for-examination-or-treatment-second-edition (accessed 17 October 2013).

Department of Health (DH). 2012. *Transforming Care: A National Response to Winterbourne View Hospital.* Available from: https://www.gov.uk/government/uploads/system/uploads/attachment_data/file/213215/final-report.pdf (accessed 17 October 2013).

Disability Discrimination Act. 1995. http://www.legislation.gov.uk/ukpga/1995/50/contents (accessed 26 April 2014).

Domestic Violence, Crime and Victims Act. 2004. http://www.legislation.gov.uk/ukpga/2004/28/contents (accessed 26 April 2014).

Donoghue v. *Stevenson* [1932]. AC 562.

Equal Pay Act. 1970. http://www.legislation.gov.uk/ukpga/1970/41 (accessed 26 April 2014).

Equality Act. 2010. Available from: http://www.legislation.gov.uk/ukpga/2010/15/contents (accessed 17 October 2013).

Equality and Human Rights Commission (EHRC). 2012. *Human Rights Review 2012: How Fair Is Britain? An Assessment of How Well Public Authorities Protect Human Rights*. EHRC. Available from: http://www.equalityhumanrights.com/uploaded_files/ehrc_full_document210312.pdf (accessed 17 October 2013).

European Convention on Human Rights. 1950. http://www.echr.coe.int/Documents/Convention_ENG.pdf (accessed 26 April 2014).

Gallagher, A., Hodge, S. (eds.). 2012. *Ethics, Law and Professional Issues. A Practical-Based Approach for Health Professionals*. Basingstoke, UK: Palgrave Macmillan.

Herring, J. 2013. *Medical Law*. Harlow, UK: Pearson Education.

Human Rights Act. 1998. Available from: http://www.legislation.gov.uk/ukpga/1998/42/introduction (accessed 17 October 2013).

Jackson, E. 2010. *Medical Law Text, Cases and Materials*. 2nd edn. Oxford: Oxford University Press.

Laming, W.H. 2003. *The Victoria Climbié Inquiry*. Available from: http://www.official-documents.gov.uk/document/cm57/5730/5730.pdf (accessed 17 October 2013).

McHale, J., Fox, M. 2006. *Health Care Law. Texts and Materials*. 2nd edn. London: Sweet & Maxwell.

Mental Capacity Act. 2005. Available from: http://www.legislation.gov.uk/ukpga/2005/9/section/22 (accessed 17 October 2013).

Mental Health Act. 1983. http://www.legislation.gov.uk/ukpga/1983/20/contents (accessed 26 April 2014).

Mental Health Act. 2007. http://www.legislation.gov.uk/ukpga/2007/12/contents (accessed 26 April 2014).

Ministry of Justice. 2006. *Human Rights: Human Lives. A Handbook for Public Authorities*. Available from: http://www.justice.gov.uk/downloads/human-rights/human-rights-handbook-for-public-authorities.pdf (accessed September 2013).

Race Relations Act. 1976. http://www.legislation.gov.uk/ukpga/1976/74 (accessed 26 April 2014).

Re C (Adult: Refusal of Treatment) [1994]. 1 All ER 819.

Re T (Adult: Refusal of Treatment) [1992]. All ER 649.

Savage v. *South Essex Partnership NHS Foundation Trust* [2010]. EWHC 865 (QB) (28 April 2010).

Scottish Human Rights Commission (SHRC). 2009. *Human Rights in a Health Care Setting: Making It Work for Everyone, An Evaluation of a Human Rights-Based Approach at the State Hospital*. Available from: http://www.scottishhumanrights.com/application/resources/documents/SHRCHealthCare.pdf (accessed 17 October 2013).

Sex Discrimination Act. 1975. http://www.legislation.gov.uk/ukpga/1975/65 (accessed 26 April 2014).

Stauch, M., Wheat, K., Tingle, J. 2002. *Sourcebook on Medical Law.* 2nd edn. London: Cavendish Publishing Limited.

6

Dignity and nursing practice

Introduction

Dignity is a human right and is important to every individual but can become compromised during health care. Being treated with dignity and involved in decision-making is associated with positive outcomes, such as high patient satisfaction (Beach et al. 2005). In a review of the general population surveys of the World Health Organisation (WHO) in 41 countries, most participants selected dignity as the second most important domain in care; only 'promptness of care' was more highly rated (Valentine et al. 2008). There are continuing concerns, however, that not all patients have dignified care experiences, with particular concerns raised about dignity of older people (House of Lords/House of Commons 2007; Health Service Ombudsman 2011) and people with learning disabilities (Mencap 2012; Care Quality Commission [CQC] 2012). Even though all National Health Service (NHS) staff have a duty to treat people with dignity, nurses are the largest group of healthcare professionals and are with patients when they are at their most vulnerable. Therefore, nurses have a major influence on whether patients feel that their dignity is preserved during their care.

Learning outcomes

By the end of this chapter, you will be able to

- Recognise legal, professional and health policy perspectives on dignity in care;
- Discuss the meaning of dignity and how the promotion or loss of dignity affects the experience of care;
- Analyse influences on dignity: the complexity of dignity, vulnerability of health service users, care environment, and attitudes, interactions and communication;
- Reflect on how nurses can promote dignity in practice for people across the lifespan and in different care settings.

Professional, legal and health policy perspectives on dignity in care

As Figure 6.1 portrays, there are professional, legal, and health policy expectations that nurses will promote dignity in nursing practice. All nurses have a professional duty to promote the dignity of those in their care. The International Council of Nurses' *Code of Ethics for Nurses* (2012) sets out that 'inherent in nursing is respect for human rights, including the right to life, to dignity and to be treated with respect'. In the United Kingdom, the Code of the Nursing and Midwifery Council (NMC) states that nurses must 'make the care of people your first concern, treating them as individuals and respecting their dignity' (NMC 2008, p. 2). As explored in Chapter 2, as a student nurse, you are expected to work within the Code.

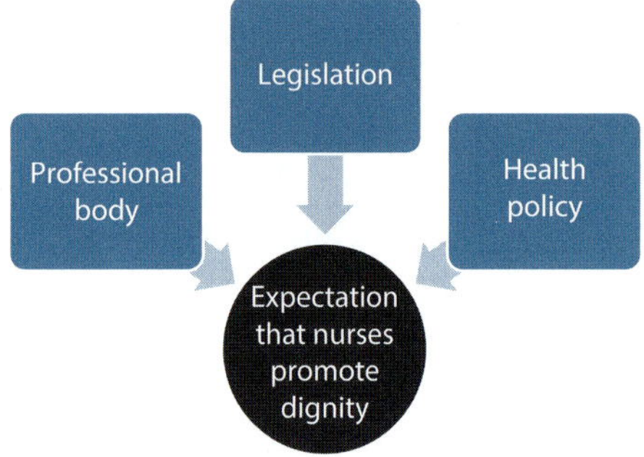

Figure 6.1 Expectations that nurses will promote dignity during care.

The Amsterdam Declaration recognised dignity as one of the main rights for patients (WHO 1994). The Human Rights Act (HRA) (1998) of the United Kingdom established that all individuals have minimal and fundamental human rights. Chapter 5 explains the HRA in detail; two of the articles are particularly relevant to dignity in health care:

- Article 3, 'Prohibition of Torture': 'No one should be subjected to torture or to inhuman or degrading treatment or punishment'. The Francis Inquiry (2013) into care at the Mid-Staffordshire NHS Foundation Trust provided numerous examples of patients subjected to degradation (e.g. left naked and covered in faeces).
- Article 8, 'Right to Respect for Private and Family Life': 'Everyone has the right to respect for his private and family life, his home and his correspondence'. Privacy is closely aligned with dignity (see further discussion in this chapter), and provision of privacy in health care, including confidentiality, is a key principle in professional practice.

Health policy documents increasingly emphasise the importance of compassionate and dignified care. The NHS Constitution (Department of Health [DH] 2013) includes 'respect and dignity' as one of the seven NHS values. The National Institute for Health and Clinical Excellence (NICE) quality standard on service user experience in adult mental health in the NHS in England includes the following standard: 'People using mental health services, and their families or carers, feel they are treated with empathy, dignity and respect' (NICE 2011, p. 7). The quality standard for care of adults in the hospital states that all staff involved in providing NHS services should 'treat patients with respect, kindness, dignity, compassion, understanding, courtesy and honesty' (NICE 2012, p. 8).

The meaning of dignity

The previous section established that from legal, health policy and professional perspectives, nurses should provide care with dignity. However, although the word *dignity* is frequently used, particularly in relation to health care, it is often not defined and has been described as an ambiguous, vague concept (Tadd et al. 2002; Macklin 2003).

Activity

Reflect on the following questions:

- What is dignity?
- How does it feel to have your dignity?
- How does it feel to lose your dignity?
- Now, ask someone else for their views and compare these with your own.

Dignity is a complex concept; in 2008, the Royal College of Nursing (RCN) published a working definition, based on a literature review, to guide nursing practice (see Box 6.1). How does this compare with your ideas? The definition emphasises that dignity applies to people whether they have capacity or not. This statement refers to mental capacity, which you explored in Chapter 5 with regard to the Mental Capacity Act. In relation to dignity loss, those most vulnerable may well be people who lack capacity to independently make their own decisions, for example, a person who is unconscious or has advanced dementia or a severe learning disability.

There are many interpretations of dignity; these are based on theories, concept analyses, and primary research conducted with patients, families

Box 6.1

Definition of dignity

Dignity is concerned with how people feel, think and behave in relation to the worth or value of themselves and others. To treat someone with dignity is to treat them as being of worth in a way that is respectful of them as valued individuals. When dignity is present, people feel in control, valued, confident, comfortable and able to make decisions for themselves. When dignity is absent people feel devalued, lacking control and comfort. They may lack confidence and be unable to make decisions for themselves. They may feel humiliated, embarrassed or ashamed. Dignity applies equally to those who have capacity and to those who lack it. Everyone has equal worth as human beings and must be treated as if they are able to feel, think and behave in relation to their own worth or value.

From Royal College of Nursing (RCN). 2008. *Defending Dignity—Challenges and Opportunities*. London: RCN, p. 8. Reproduced with permission from Royal College of Nursing.

and healthcare professionals. Some of these views are discussed next. As you read the material, consider also how these views relate to your own ideas.

Nordenfelt (2003) examined the meaning of dignity and identified four types:

- *menschenwűrde* (the dignity that all humans have equally);
- merit (because of position in society or earned through achievements);
- moral stature (because of moral deeds—a virtue);
- dignity of identity (integrity of body and mind).

Primary research studies based in health care (Matiti 2002; Jacelon 2003) and concept analyses of dignity (Jacelon et al. 2004; Griffin-Heslin 2005; Jacobson, 2007) all support the notion of human dignity. However, Nordenfelt's (2003) concept of dignity as merit or moral stature is of questionable relevance in health care. Chapter 1 discussed non-discriminatory behaviour in nursing practice; all patients should be treated equally with respect for their dignity, regardless of perceived merit or moral status (Baillie 2009). Nordenfelt's (2003) fourth type of dignity, dignity as personal identity, is readily applicable to health care as illness and disability may threaten personal identity through the impact on body image (Lin and Tsai 2011) and mental and physical ability (Baillie 2009). For example, a patient being treated for cancer may lose his or her hair and might need help with personal care because of the debilitating effect of the condition and treatment. This person could experience these effects as detrimental to personal identity and as a threat to dignity.

In another analysis of dignity, Jacobson (2007) proposed two categories:

- human dignity: the dignity that all humans have;
- social dignity: experienced through interaction; the dignity of self and dignity in relation to others.

Jacobson (2007) argued that although human dignity cannot be taken away, social dignity is affected by our interactions with ourselves and with others and, as such, can be threatened or lost. Following from her analysis, with all patients we care for we must acknowledge and respect their human dignity and recognise that dignity relates to how they feel, their relationships and their interactions. Their social dignity will be affected by their interactions with their families and friends and with other patients in a ward situation, as well as with the healthcare workers. Baillie (2009) found that patients had a mainly positive effect on the dignity of each other as they felt comforted that other patients were 'in the same boat' as themselves and by the care and concern shown to each other. You might consider, then, the effect on dignity when patients who have formed supportive relationships are moved around and between wards. In Slettebø et al.'s (2009) study, patients specifically referred to support from family and friends as a factor that preserved their dignity during rehabilitation. Therefore, people at home or in hospital who have no visitors and few people to interact with, may be more vulnerable to diminished dignity. Interactions with healthcare staff then become even more important in relation to their dignity.

Key features of dignity in health care

From reviewing a range of theories, concept analyses and primary research about dignity, Matiti and Baillie (2011) summarised some key features of dignity with reference to health care:

- Dignity is inherent to being a human being.
- Dignity is dynamic; for example, patients adjust their perceptions of dignity during hospitalisation and as illness progresses.
- Dignity is an internal quality: an aspect of self that is closely linked to each person's individuality, feelings and uniqueness.
- Dignity relates to feelings such as self-esteem, self-worth, pride, confidence, feeling important and valuable and feeling comfortable.

- Dignity relates to behaviour, for example, behaving according to one's personal standards, behaving courteously, showing mutual respect, and treating people as individuals and as important and valuable.
- Dignity concerns relationships: interpersonal dignity and relationships involving reciprocal behaviour.
- Control is important for dignity; related concepts are autonomy and independence.
- Presentation of self (e.g. physical appearance) in public is important for many people's dignity.
- Privacy is important, including personal space, privacy of the body and privacy of personal information (confidentiality).

Review the scenario in Box 6.2 and the questions that follow. We refer to Hanna's scenario further in this chapter as we discuss dignity in care.

Box 6.2

Practice scenario: a visit to the Children's Assessment Unit

Hanna is 4 months old and over several days became 'chesty': coughing and wheezing and 'struggling to breathe'. She also had a raised temperature. Having rang the out-of-hours general practitioner service, Hanna was referred to the Children's Assessment Unit at a local hospital. The family was shown into a crowded waiting room. A pleasant nurse took details and recorded some observations, but Hanna's parents felt embarrassed about disclosing private information in front of the other parents. They were asked to collect a urine sample from Hanna, a 'clean catch'. This meant that Hanna had to sit on her mother's lap without a nappy over a plastic pot until she passed urine. Hanna's mother felt uncomfortable that Hanna was exposed to a room of strangers. When the urine sample test had been done, the nurse told the result to another mother by mistake. Hanna's parents felt dismayed by this lack of care.

After a couple of hours, Hanna needed feeding. When her mother asked for somewhere private to breastfeed, the response was dismissive: raised eyebrows and a curt 'there isn't anywhere' before grudgingly showing Hanna and her mother an office to use. Hours went by without any communication about why the wait to see the doctor was so long or any inquiry about how Hanna was or whether she or her parents needed anything.

Questions

1. How do you think Hanna's parents might have felt in this situation? Look again at the RCN's definition of dignity in Box 6.1 and consider the impact on dignity.
2. Look at the key features of dignity in health care: How do these relate to Hanna and her parents?

Influences on dignity in care

Figure 6.2 portrays the influences on dignity in care and highlights the complexity involved in ensuring that all patients have dignified care experiences all of the time in all care settings. Dignity is a multi-faceted concept, and the dignity of people accessing health care is further affected by their own personal factors and vulnerabilities, including their mental and physical health; the care environment, which in the hospital includes not only their bed space on a ward but also different departments they might visit for treatment or investigations and even the corridors and lift; and all the different interactions they have with both clinical and non-clinical staff, with other patients and their families.

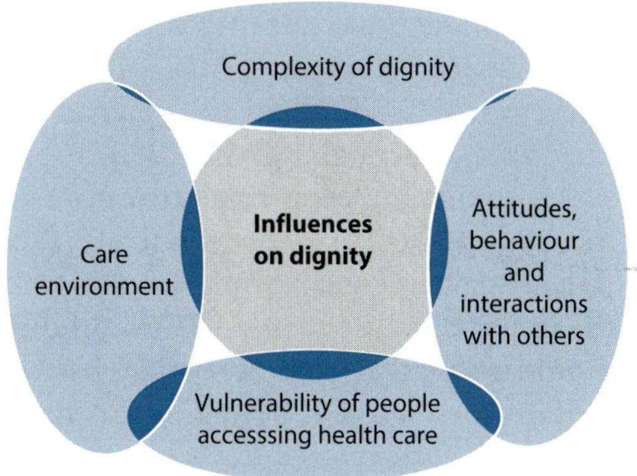

Figure 6.2 Influences on dignity in care.

In a study of UK nurses' strategies to promote dignity in practice, Baillie and Gallagher (2011) identified five core elements that applied across all care settings: recognising vulnerability to dignity loss; enhancing privacy; improving communication between staff and patients/families and building relationships; improving the care environment; and addressing issues that matter to individuals. Baillie and Gallagher found that nurses applied these core elements to their own particular setting, and they recommended that nurses should identify and address dignity issues specific to their own practice areas. As an example, in the scenario in Box 6.2, nurses on the Children's Assessment Unit should recognise the vulnerability of young children and their parents, who will feel anxious and lacking control. The nurses could have ensured that they gave privacy whilst taking personal details, kept the families informed about what was happening when they were waiting to be seen by the doctor, and offered a private room for breastfeeding.

Complexity of dignity

Figure 6.3 portrays the complex and fragile nature of dignity, which means that promoting a person's dignity is multi-faceted and an ongoing process. Dignity is not a static phenomenon but is dynamic and can fluctuate, affected by interactions, events, the person's own feelings and care environment factors. Looking back at the scenario in Box 6.2, you can see how the series of events might have gradually diminished the dignity of Hanna and her parents. Consider also how a person's individuality might affect the person's dignity. Baillie (2007a) found that for some patients, having some control, however small, was the most important influencing factor for their dignity (e.g. having some choice over what was happening to them). However, for other patients, physical presentation was particularly important; for example, one woman said, in relation to her dignity, that she would never go out without her make-up and always dressed 'nicely'. Accordingly, following her bed bath she asked for her make-up bag and mirror so that she could apply her make-up, later asking whether her lipstick was on straight (Baillie 2007a, p. 124). For other patients, privacy was the most important aspect, and some patients found being in a hospital bay with other patients incompatible with dignity. However, other patients gained comfort and support from being in a bay with patients with similar conditions and did not find it an undignified experience. We should recognise, therefore, that patients' views about what is most important for their dignity might vary and differ from our own views.

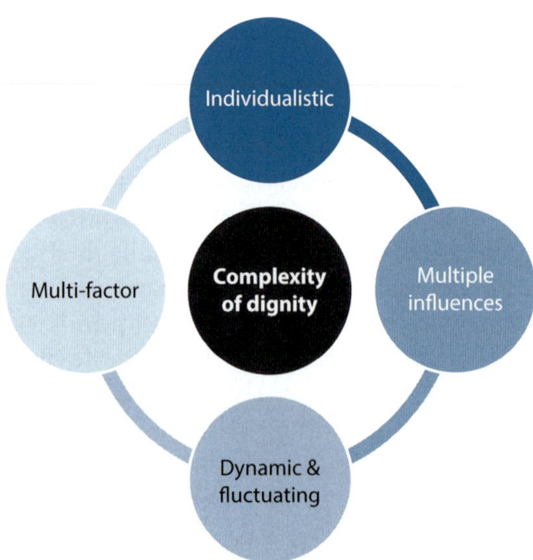

Figure 6.3 The complexity of dignity.

Activity

Reflect on what is most important for your own dignity. If you were attending hospital for an outpatient appointment:

- What would be the top three factors that would help preserve your dignity in this situation?
- What would be the top three factors that would diminish your dignity in an outpatient setting?

Ask a friend or family member these questions and compare the answers to your own. Were your views the same or different?

Vulnerability of people accessing health care

There are many factors that can increase vulnerability to loss of dignity; we explore them in this section.

Activity

Reflect on a recent healthcare experience in a specific care setting, as a student, a patient or a relative. What specific factors would make patients in this setting vulnerable to dignity loss?

Specific factors that increase vulnerability to a loss of dignity include life stage, the effect of health conditions, and negative attitudes and stigma. The factors you identified might have related to one or more of these factors. Human beings, when ill or during life-stage processes, may experience changes in themselves that can threaten their dignity (Matiti and Baillie 2011). Health conditions can affect people's identity through an impact on body image or function, and during health care, people often experience discomfort and a loss of control and confidence. In Berg and Danielson's (2007) study, in relation to dignity, patients with severe and acute long-term illnesses talked of feeling 'so small and so vulnerable'.

Life-stage effects on dignity

Much of the media attention on indignity has centred on older people, who are the core users of adult health services. Older people are particularly likely to have co-morbidities, and growing numbers have dementia, as this is associated with ageing. Such were the concerns about lack of dignity for older people in hospitals and care homes that a commission was set up to investigate the situation (Commission on Dignity in Care 2012). The commission's report comprehensively reviewed evidence, both shortcomings and good practices, and included many recommendations to address the dignity of older people. However, dignity is important to people across the lifespan.

Reed (2011) asserted that dignity for children is often overlooked and is sometimes considered of less value or relevance than dignity of adults. In her research, a nurse commented that the view is often: 'They are only babies, so people think it doesn't matter' (p. 89). If you look again at Box 6.2, you might notice the nurse's expectation that Hanna should be exposed in a crowded waiting room to collect the urine sample. Reed (2011) pointed out the vulnerability of babies as they are small, unable to move about, cannot communicate their needs verbally and their daily needs have to be met through another. She further highlighted that children often lack power, control and involvement in decision-making. Burden (2011) explored how women's dignity can be affected during pregnancy and childbirth, with particular reference to privacy aspects but also that they lack control over what is happening to them much of the time. The need for dignity at the end of life is well recognised; indeed, a number of research studies have identified dignity as one of the most important issues in end-of-life care (Vohra et al. 2004; Touhy et al. 2005; Aspinal et al. 2006).

How physical and mental health affect dignity

Physical and mental health status can affect dignity in many ways. Baillie (2009) found that patients' impaired health led to dependence in personal care, which threatened dignity. Dementia affects independence in many daily activities, such as in the abilities to communicate, eat and drink, move around safely, make decisions, and carry out personal care. Baillie (2009) also found that a serious illness, or uncertainty about diagnosis, led to patients feeling out of control, which diminished their dignity.

Specific attributes of many health conditions increase vulnerability to indignity. In Baillie and Gallagher's (2011) study, nurses identified that conditions affecting physical appearance and body image affected patients' dignity. For example, a staff nurse on a ward that dealt with head and neck cancer considered that there were

> *so many issues with regards to dignity, loads of facial disfigurement, body image issues, people not able to eat, people not able to speak, not able to kiss*
> *(Baillie and Gallagher 2011, p. 337)*

The nurses expressed that to anticipate and minimise experiences of indignity, they needed to be sensitive to the dignity issues associated with specific health conditions whilst also addressing the issues of importance to each individual.

In another example of how specific health conditions affect dignity, Baillie (2007b) reported on how urological conditions detracted from dignity. Some patients felt embarrassed about their diagnosis, and the associated intimate examinations and treatments diminished dignity for some people. Some patients could rationalise having to have a urinary catheter, but for others it presented a total lack of dignity. Urinary incontinence, which was also associated with indignity (Baillie 2007b), is common among the population. Estimated prevalence increases with age (DH 2000), and incontinence is often associated with other conditions, particularly those affecting mobility (Chiarelli and Weatherall 2010). Therefore, incontinence can be another factor compounding vulnerability to dignity loss.

Mental health conditions can affect dignity, partly because of the associated stigma and discrimination service users face, and the nature of mental health care environments (see further sections). Stacey and Stickley (2011) highlighted the vulnerability of people who have experienced years of mental health problems and the social consequences, who then become older and also develop physical health conditions. They argued that when physical frailty is accompanied with mental frailty, the individual's dignity is at greatest risk.

Stigma and discrimination

Jacobson (2009) identified discriminatory behaviour as a dignity violation. As discussed in Chapter 1, health professionals are legally and professionally required to behave in an anti-discriminatory manner, but discrimination in health care is often reported and may be individual, institutional or societal (Baillie and Matiti 2013). Baillie and Matiti (2013) explored discrimination in health care in relation to age, disability and sexuality, and the effects on dignity, arguing that a person-centred approach to care can promote dignity by responding to and valuing diversity of individuals. Many people experience stigma or discrimination in their day-to-day lives, which may affect their confidence and self-esteem, so when they access health care, they already feel vulnerable. People who are diagnosed with a mental health problem often report that they experience 'a downward spiral of loss, social disadvantage and isolation' (Stacey and Stickley 2011, p. 175). The Royal College of Psychiatrists (2013) reported that people with mental health problems frequently experience stigma and discrimination, not only in the wider community but also from services. Specifically, people with dementia may face stigma and discrimination in society and health care (Chan and Chan 2009). Stacey and Stickley (2011) argued that care workers in mental health must tackle the stigma and subsequent discrimination associated with mental health problems if they are to promote recovery.

Hallawell (2011) highlighted that historically, people with learning disabilities have experienced breaches of their dignity, which continue to this day, despite the HRA (1998) and the Equality Act (2010). Various reports highlighted the experiences of indignity in care, with many of these experiences revealing discriminatory behaviour (Mencap 2004, 2007, 2012). Other examples of people whose dignity is at risk because of stigma are bariatric (morbidly obese) patients. Thomas and Lee-Fong (2010) highlighted prevailing negative attitudes towards people who are bariatric and the humiliating situations that some patients face. They argue for education of health professionals about caring for people who are bariatric and for healthcare organisations to have protocols and resources in place.

As this section has explained, people accessing health care are vulnerable to dignity loss for multiple reasons. However, staff behaviour and the care environment can do much to promote dignity.

Attitudes, behaviour and interactions with others

Widäng and Fridlund (2003) argued that promoting dignity is dependent on how patients are treated by their caregivers. There are three key aspects of staff behaviour that affect dignity in care: interactions and communication; provision of privacy; and essential care. The attitudes of staff affect how the behaviour is carried out and how it is perceived. For example, in Bayer et al.'s (2005) study, older people considered that attitudes of caregivers were central to dignified care, as attitudes could portray that the person is valued. In the scenario in Box 6.2, the nurse found a private room for Hanna's mother to breastfeed, but the nurse's attitude diminished dignity, portraying a lack of respect and sensitivity. Baillie and Gallagher (2011) found that treating people as valued individuals was the core factor that promoted dignity.

Interactions and communication

A key aspect of promoting dignity is about getting to know a person and developing a relationship with them through your interactions. For people with communication difficulties, you will need to use creative ways and work closely with families. As an example, the Alzheimer's Society's 'This Is Me' leaflet is increasingly being filled in with people with dementia and their families, as a way of communicating their preferences, likes and dislikes (see http://www.alzheimers.org.uk/site/scripts/documents_info.php?documentID=1290). Similarly, people with learning disabilities should have a communication passport or comparable document.

Non-verbal communication is as important as verbal in interactions that influence dignity. For example, in a study of older people's transitions between care services, Ellins et al. (2012) noted the following:

> *One of the most striking findings was that even the smallest gestures by providers to connect with somebody as a human being—such as a smile or a hug—could make a significant difference to their sense of dignity and their experience overall.*
>
> *(Ellins et al. 2012, p. 131)*

Communication that promotes dignity helps people to feel comfortable, in control and valued (see Table 6.1).

Table 6.1 Interactions that Make Patients Feel Comfortable, In Control and Valued

Interactions that help people feel comfortable	• Sensitivity
	• Empathy
	• Developing relationships
	• Conversation
	• Professionalism
	• Family involvement (if desired by the patient)
	• Friendliness and reassurance
	• Humour (if used sensitively and appropriately)
Communication that helps people feel in control	• Giving explanations and information
	• Providing informed consent
	• Offering choices and negotiating
	• Enabling independence
Communication that helps people to feel valued	• Listening
	• Giving time
	• Showing concern for patients as individuals
	• Being kind, considerate and helpful
	• Showing courtesy: addressing people by their preferred name, introducing self, being polite and respectful, including respect for culture and religious beliefs

Source: Adapted from Baillie, L. 2007. A case study of patient dignity in an acute hospital setting. Unpublished thesis. London South Bank University, Royal College of Nursing (RCN). 2008. *Defending Dignity—Challenges and Opportunities*. London: RCN.

In Baillie's (2009) study, interactions that diminished dignity were found to be curtness (being brusque or offhand) and being authoritarian, with one patient saying:

> *It's like you're a thing in a bed and I'm coming round. You have to have all these tablets whether you want them or not.*
>
> *(p. 31)*

Jacobson (2009) focussed specifically on behaviours that violated patients' dignity, most of which are interactions: rudeness; indifference; condescension (talking down to); dismissal (when practitioners discount patients' concerns, needs, feelings etc.); disregard (e.g. ignoring); dependence (because of the patient's condition but exacerbated by practitioners' attitudes); intrusion (breaching privacy); objectification (treated as a 'thing' not a person); restriction (of movement, access to belongings); labelling (e.g. as 'difficult'); contempt (treated without value); discrimination; revulsion; deprivation (e.g. preventing access to necessities); assault and abjection (being forced to compromise one's beliefs).

Activity

Consider the behaviours that violate dignity, as outlined previously:

- Reflect on your practice experience: Have you witnessed any of these behaviours?
- How would you respond if you observed staff behaviour that violated dignity?

Chapter 11 addresses in detail how to raise concerns about care, and these could include staff behaviour that violates dignity. It is also important to restore dignity for patients sensitively and promptly.

Providing privacy

There are three key areas of privacy for people accessing health care: privacy of personal space, privacy of their bodies and confidentiality. Whilst the care environment influences privacy, staff behaviour strongly affects experiences of privacy; see the work of Baillie (2011) for a detailed overview of privacy provision in different care settings. Individual staff behaviour to provide privacy is strongly influenced by the care culture and values (see Chapter 1).

As regards personal space, some studies have found that in hospital, patients' personal territory, their bed space and locker, were not respected by staff (Matiti 2002; Woogara 2004). Patients may feel that their personal space has been breached when staff move patients' belongings around in their bedside lockers or other furniture without discussion or when staff enter closed curtains or doors without asking. In community-based care, staff should only enter areas of a person's home that are necessary for carrying out care, always checking with the person first. In a hospital setting, nurses should close doors or fully draw bedside curtains when privacy is needed, preferably applying a 'Do not disturb' notice or a peg to curtains to deter intrusion. In hospital bays, patients should always be taken to the toilet or bathroom, if their medical condition permits, rather than having personal care at the bedside.

People undergoing health care are at risk of bodily exposure as they often need to undress for procedures or examinations and need help with personal care. There are research reports of staff exposing people's bodies and being inattentive to their privacy (Woolhead et al. 2005; Matiti 2002) and of staff intrusion behind curtains during intimate procedures involving bodily exposure (Ariño-Blasco et al. 2005; Baillie 2009). Other examples of privacy breaches are bedside curtains that are not fully closed during personal care, removal of clothing without discussion or consent, or providing clothing that does not cover patients' bodies adequately (e.g. hospital gowns that do not close fully at the back) (Baillie 2009). Sometimes, traditional practices have led to patients being expected to undress into nightclothes or hospital gowns long before it is necessary and for staff convenience, rather than patients' well-being. People undergoing health care should dress in their own clothes as much as possible; if they have to wear nightclothes, provide dressing gowns for them when sitting out of bed or moving around. When hospital gowns are used for operations or examinations, ensure that they are fastened properly; look for newer styles that are less exposing. If patients are sitting outside the room or being taken somewhere in a wheelchair, they must be adequately covered so that their bodies are not exposed. When a patient's body is exposed for a procedure or examination, only the minimum clothing should be removed, ensuring that the rest of the patient's body is covered by bed linen or clothing. Some patients will not wish to expose their bodies to staff of the opposite sex; religious beliefs may influence individual views about modesty. Nurses should behave sensitively and respect people's wishes.

Maintaining privacy of information (confidentiality) is another staff behaviour that promotes dignity (Calnan et al. 2005; Matiti 2002). As discussed in Chapter 2, confidentiality has legal and professional dimensions. Lack of confidentiality occurs when personal information (e.g. about incontinence, medical diagnosis or home circumstances) is overheard or displayed in public areas. Most health and social care organisations have confidentiality policies that provide specific guidance about information giving. In curtained areas in the hospital, curtains provide a visual barrier, but auditory privacy is more difficult. If exposing or intimate procedures have to be carried out at the bedside, staff should communicate discreetly, by keeping voices low and using non-verbal communication. Staff should ensure that patients with hearing impairments have working hearing aids in place and that they maintain good face-to-face contact to better enable lip-reading.

Essential care

Essential care is the personal care that most people can carry out for themselves independently from early childhood, including personal hygiene, dressing, going to the toilet and eating and drinking. Personal care is essential for health and comfort and has an impact on dignity through effects on self-esteem and confidence. We all have our individual standards and preferred ways of carrying out personal care; these are part of our personal identity and therefore our dignity. Unfortunately, there are many reports of dignity being diminished by poor-quality personal care (Patients Association 2009; Francis Inquiry 2013); in such situations, patients will feel uncomfortable, uncared for and unvalued as well as experience incontinence, hunger, thirst, pain and poor hygiene.

To promote dignity, essential care must be delivered to a high standard, with privacy and communication that promotes dignity. The *Essence of Care* (DH 2010) provides benchmarks for best practice in essential care: bladder, bowel and continence care; food and drink; prevention and management of pain; personal hygiene; and prevention and management of pressure ulcers, as well as other important care areas. The book *Developing Practical Nursing Skills* (Baillie 2014) explains essential care in detail and is recommended further reading.

In practice, you may care for some people who appear reluctant for you to carry out essential care; you should approach each person as an individual to address their needs appropriately. Read the practice scenario in Box 6.3 and reflect on the questions posed. You may wish to refer to the information about the Mental Capacity Act in Chapter 5 when considering John's capacity to make decisions about his personal care.

Box 6.3

Practice scenario: personal care and dignity

John, a widower, has advanced dementia and is a resident in a care home. His daughter, Catherine, visits him most evenings after work. On several occasions, she has found him unshaven and wearing soiled clothes from the previous day, with dried-on food. She feels upset as her father was always meticulous about personal hygiene, had a daily shave and was smartly dressed. She raised her concerns about his personal care with the care home manager, who checked John's care record. She told Catherine that John sometimes refuses a wash and shave and that the care workers therefore respect his decision.

Questions

1. How might a lack of personal care for John affect his dignity?
2. Does John have the mental capacity to make his own decision about his personal care?
3. How else could care home staff approach such situations?

It is likely that John's daughter knows his preferences and what is important for her father's personal identity, as well as for his comfort. Choice and control are important for dignity but under the Mental Capacity Act 2005, John may not have the capacity to make decisions about his personal care, and staff should act in his best interests. However, John may have capacity to decide if the choice is conveyed to him in a different way. Because of the memory problems associated with dementia, John may not recognise the vocabulary associated with personal care. The carers might have had a different response had they shown John his shaving and washing equipment and some alternative clean clothes, rather than using verbal communication alone. They could have returned later with a fresh approach and asked him in a different way. The Alzheimer's Society provides useful guides, such as 'Top Tips for Nurses' (see http://www.alzheimers.org.uk/site/scripts/documents_info.php?documentID=1211), which they developed in response to research about concerns of nurses and carers; you should find these helpful in practice when caring for a person with dementia.

Healthcare staff attitudes, behaviour and interactions have a major influence on dignity in care but should not be seen in isolation from the care environment, particularly the care culture, and this dimension is explored next.

Care environment

The next activity will prompt you to explore how the care environment affects dignity.

Activity

Consider healthcare environments you have encountered, as a patient, relative or in practice learning experiences.

- What aspects helped dignity? What aspects threatened dignity? Think about the whole care environment, not just the physical aspects.
- Return to Box 6.2. Can you identify any environmental factors that influenced the dignity of Hanna and her parents?

Baillie (2009) identified that the physical environment, organisational culture, leadership and healthcare systems are components of the care environment that influence dignity. In Box 6.2, the Children's Assessment Unit apparently provided little privacy for children and their families waiting for assessment. However, you might also consider the culture of this environment. Hanna's mother was treated with disdain when she asked for somewhere private to breastfeed but an empty office was then grudgingly found for her. Chapter 1 explores how the values of organisations and individual units influence the culture and individual behaviour, much depending on leadership.

The recent reports into poor care at Winterbourne View Hospital (DH 2012) and the Mid Staffordshire NHS Foundation Trust (Francis 2013) both highlighted that the culture of an organisation influences whether compassionate and dignified care is provided. The culture of an organisation also influences the systems put in place, affecting whether people feel treated as an individual or a number. Baillie and Illott (2010) gave the example of a patient left to wait on a trolley for a long time outside the operating theatre as the anaesthetist was apparently double-booked. The patient described the impact on her dignity:

> *It just makes you aware that you are patient number nine hundred and fifty nine and you don't matter You're in a meat market. And you're on a conveyor belt.*
>
> *(p. 279)*

Reports have highlighted frequent, disorientating and undignifying moves for patients between hospital wards, particularly for older people (Royal College of Physicians 2012; Cornwell et al. 2012). Research exploring the views of people who use mental health services has found that people often feel stripped of dignity in the mental health system (Stacey and Stickley 2011).

The physical environment includes aspects such as privacy (e.g. reasonable bed space size, well-fitting bed curtains, space for private conversations, sufficient bathrooms and toilets). A clean environment with good standards of décor is also important, as it is demeaning (as well as hazardous) for people to be cared for in unclean, neglected environments. Mixed-sex accommodation has been found to diminish patients' dignity in acute hospitals (Baillie 2008) and also has a detrimental effect within mental health wards (Stacey and Stickley 2011). UK health policy directives now require there to be single-sex accommodation, defined as single-sex sleeping and bathroom facilities, with certain exceptions (e.g. critical care) (DH 2011).

In the past, people with learning disabilities experienced particularly undignifying care environments: impoverished with little or no privacy; institutions situated at a distance from the person's home, family and friends; restricted or no access to the outside world; and all resources, activities and experiences supplied within the institution (RCN 2010). When caring for older people with learning disabilities, you might remember that much of their lives could have been spent in such environments. Much progress has been made, with a move towards people with learning disabilities living independently in the community or in supported housing. However, the recent scandal of the Winterbourne View Hospital for people with learning disabilities, where residents often came from long distances away and experienced neglectful and abusive care, highlighted that inappropriate environments for people with learning disabilities have not been eliminated (DH 2012).

In Baillie and Gallagher's (2011) study, nurses explained the environmental changes they were making to improve dignity. These included making care home bedroom doors more like an apartment entrance and developing facilities for relatives of intensive therapy unit patients. A stroke unit Sister described enhanced bathroom facilities so that patients could be wheeled into the bathroom for undressing, as previously, through lack of space, patients were dressed and undressed at the bedside and taken to the bathroom wrapped in sheets. A dementia unit manager described how a nurse was individualizing the environment, so that 'every single room looks as if that's just their room and nobody else's' (p. 339). In a care home, the dining area was made to be 'more like a restaurant', offering a choice of ways to assist residents at mealtimes, ensuring meals were not disturbed, and that plates are warm. These examples illustrate how nurses can be proactive and influence the environment to promote dignity in care.

Chapter summary

Dignity is a human right and is important to every individual but can become compromised during health care. This chapter reviewed legal, professional and health policy perspectives that confirmed the duty of nurses to promote the dignity of people in their care. The meaning of dignity was explored and highlighted the complexity and multi-faceted nature of dignity. The dignity of people accessing health care is affected by their own personal factors and vulnerabilities, including their mental and physical health. Whether their dignity is lost is influenced by the care environment (physical environment, organisational culture, leadership and healthcare systems) and staff behaviour (interactions and communication; provision of privacy; and meeting essential care needs). All healthcare staff have a duty to promote dignity of patients, but nurses, who are consistently present when patients are at their most vulnerable, can make a major difference to dignity in care.

Further resources

- There is a Dignity in Care network that has a website, which provides many resources for health and social care and where you can sign up to be a dignity champion (http://www.dignityincare.org.uk). Look for the annual Dignity in Care action day, promoted on this site, and become involved if you can.

- The Social Care Institute for Excellence (SCIE) provides a series of practice guides on dignity in care (see http://www.scie.org.uk), which are a useful resource.
- In 2008–2009, the RCN ran an extensive campaign 'Dignity at the Heart of Everything We Do', and resources remain available (see http://www.rcn.org.uk/newsevents/campaigns/dignity).
- For further reading and a detailed exploration of dignity in different care settings and across the lifespan, see in *Dignity in Healthcare: A Practical Approach for Nurses and Midwives* (Matiti and Baillie 2011).

References

Ariño-Blasco, S., Tadd, W., Boix-Ferrer, J.A. 2005. Dignity and older people: The voice of professionals. *Quality in Ageing* 6(1): 30–35.

Aspinal, F., Hughes, R., Dunckley, M., Addington-Hall, J. 2006. What is important to measure in the last months and weeks of life? A modified nominal group study. *International Journal of Nursing Studies* 43(4): 393–403.

Baillie, L. 2007a. A case study of patient dignity in an acute hospital setting. Unpublished thesis. London South Bank University.

Baillie, L. 2007b. The impact of urological conditions on patients' dignity. *International Journal of Urological Nursing* 1(1): 27–35.

Baillie, L. 2008. Mixed sex wards and patient dignity: Nurses' and patients' perspectives. *British Journal of Nursing* 17(19): 1220–1225.

Baillie, L. 2009. Patient dignity in an acute hospital setting: A case study. *International Journal of Nursing Studies* 46: 22–36.

Baillie, L. 2011. Staff behaviour and attitudes which promote dignity in care. In Matiti, M.R., and Baillie, L. (eds.), *Dignity in Healthcare: A Practical Approach for Nurses and Midwives*. London: Radcliffe, 62–78.

Baillie, L. 2014. (Ed) *Developing Practical Nursing Skills*. 4th Edition. Abingdon: Taylor & Francis.

Baillie, L., Gallagher, A. 2011. Respecting dignity in care in diverse care settings: Strategies of UK nurses. *International Journal of Nursing Practice* 17: 336–341.

Baillie, L., Illott, L. 2010. Promoting the dignity of patients in perioperative practice. *Journal of Perioperative Care* 20(8): 278–282.

Baillie, L., Matiti, M.R. 2013. Dignity, equality and diversity: An exploration of how discriminatory behaviour of healthcare workers affects patient dignity. *Diversity and Equality in Health Care* 10(1): 5–12.

Bayer, T., Tadd, W., Krajcik, S. 2005. Dignity: The voice of older people. *Quality in Ageing* 6(1): 22–27.

Beach, C., Sugarman, J., Johnson, R., et al. 2005. Do patients treated with dignity report higher satisfaction, adherence and receipt of preventive care? *Annals of Family Medicine* 3(4): 331–338.

Berg, L., Danielson, E. 2007. Patients' and nurses' experiences of the caring relationship in hospital: An aware striving for trust. *Scandinavian Journal of Caring Sciences* 21: 500–506.

Burden, B. 2011. Dignity in maternity care. In Matiti, M.R., and Baillie, L. (eds.), *Dignity in Healthcare: A Practical Approach for Nurses and Midwives*. London: Radcliffe, 95–108.

Calnan. M., Woolhead, G., Dieppe, P. 2005. Views on dignity in providing health care for older people. *Nursing Times* 101(33): 38–41.

Care Quality Commission (CQC). 2012. *Learning Disabilities Services Inspection Programme: National Overview*. Available from: http://www.cqc.org.uk/sites/default/files/media/documents/cqc_ld_review_national_overview.pdf (accessed 22 June 2013).

Chan, P.A., Chan, T. 2009. The impact of discrimination against older people with dementia and its impact on student nurses' professional socialisation. *Nurse Education in Practice* 9: 221–227.

Chiarelli, P., Weatherall, M. 2010. The link between chronic conditions and urinary incontinence. *Australian and New Zealand Continence Journal* 16(1): 7–14.

Commission on Dignity in Care. 2012. *Delivering Dignity: Securing Dignity in Care for Older People in Hospitals and Care Homes*. Available from: http://www.nhsconfed.org/Publications/Documents/Delivering_Dignity_final_report150612.pdf (accessed 22 June 2013).

Cornwell, J., Levenson, R., Sonola, L., Poteliakhoff, E. 2012. *Continuity of Care for Older Hospital Patients: A Call for Action*. London: King's Fund.

Department of Health (DH). 2000. *Good Practice in Continence Services*. London: DH.

Department of Health (DH). 2010. *Essence of Care 2010*. Gateway reference 14641. London: Stationery Office.

Department of Health (DH). 2011. *What Is Government Policy around Eliminating Mixed-Sex Accommodation?* Gateway reference 15371. London: DH.

Department of Health (DH). 2012. *Winterbourne View Hospital: Department of Health Review and Response*. Gateway reference 18348. Available from: https://www.gov.uk/government/publications/winterbourne-view-hospital-department-of-health-review-and-response (accessed 22 June 2013).

Department of Health (DH). 2013. *The NHS Constitution for England*. Available from: https://www.gov.uk/government/publications/the-nhs-constitution-for-england (accessed 24 November 2013).

Ellins, J., Glasby, J., Tanner, D., et al. 2012. *Understanding and Improving Transitions of Older People: A User and Carer Centred Approach. Final Report.* NIHR SDO programme. http://www.nets.nihr.ac.uk/__data/assets/pdf_file/0008/85076/FR-08-1809-228.pdf (accessed 22 April 2014).

Equality Act. 2010. Available from: http://www.legislation.gov.uk/ukpga/2010/15/contents (accessed 22 June 2013).

Francis Inquiry. 2013. *Report of the Mid Staffordshire NHS Foundation Trust Public Inquiry*. Available from: http://www.midstaffspublicinquiry.com/report (accessed 22 June 2013).

Griffin-Heslin, V.L. 2005. An analysis of the concept dignity. *Accident and Emergency Nursing* 13(4): 251–257.

Hallawell, B. 2011. Dignity and people with learning disabilities. In Matiti, M.R., and Baillie, L. (eds.), *Dignity in Healthcare: A Practical Approach for Nurses and Midwives*. London: Radcliffe, 186–198.

Health Service Ombudsman. 2011. *Care and Compassion? Report of the Health Service Ombudsman on Ten Investigations into NHS Care of Older People*. Available from: http://www.ombudsman.org.uk/care-and-compassion/home (accessed 22 June 2013).

House of Lords/House of Commons. 2007. *Joint Committee on Human Rights—The Human Rights of Older People in Healthcare.* Eighteenth Report. Available from: http://www.publications.parliament.uk/pa/jt200607/jtselect/jtrights/156/15602.htm (accessed 22 June 2013).

Human Rights Act. 1998. c. 42. London: HMSO. Available from: http://www.legislation.gov.uk/ukpga/1998/42/contents (accessed 22 June 2013).

International Council of Nurses. 2012. *The ICN Code of Ethics for Nurses*. Available from: http://www.icn.ch/images/stories/documents/publications/free_publications/Code_of_Ethics_2012.pdf (accessed 22 June 2013).

Jacelon, C.S. 2003. The dignity of elders in acute care hospital. *Qualitative Health Research* 13(4): 543–556.

Jacelon, C.S., Connelly, T.W., Brown, R., Proulx, K., Vo, T. 2004. A concept analysis of dignity in older adults. *Journal of Advanced Nursing* 48(1): 76–83.

Jacobson, N. 2007. Dignity and health: A review. *Social Science and Medicine* 64(2): 292–302.

Jacobson, N. 2009. Dignity violation in healthcare. *Qualitative Health Research* 19(11): 1536–1547.

Lin, Y.P., Tsai, Y.F. 2011. Maintaining patients' dignity during clinical care: A qualitative interview study. *Journal of Advanced Nursing* 67(2): 340–348.

Macklin, R. 2003. Dignity is a useless concept: It means no more than respect for persons or their autonomy. *British Medical Journal* 327(7429): 1419–1420.

Matiti, M.R. 2002. Patient dignity in nursing: A phenomenological study. Unpublished thesis. University of Huddersfield School of Education and Professional Development.

Matiti, M.R., Baillie, L. 2011. The concept of dignity. In Matiti, M.R., and Baillie, L. (eds.), *Dignity in Health Care for Nurses and Midwives: A Practical Approach for Nurses and Midwives*. London: Radcliffe, 9–23.

Mencap. 2004. *Treat Me Right! Better Healthcare for People with a Learning Disability*. London: Mencap.

Mencap. 2007. *Death by Indifference: Following up the Treat Me Right! Report*. London: Mencap.

Mencap. 2012. *Death by Indifference: 74 Deaths and Counting: A Progress Report 5 Years On*. London: Mencap.

National Institute for Health and Clinical Excellence. 2011. *Service user experience in adult mental health: Improving the experience of care for people using adult NHS mental health services*. Clinical Guideline 136. London: NICE.

National Institute for Health and Clinical Excellence (NICE). 2012. *Patient Experience in Adult NHS Services: Improving the Experience of Care for People Using Adult NHS Services*. Clinical Guideline 138. London: NICE.

Nursing and Midwifery Council (NMC). 2008. *The Code: Standards of Conduct, Performance and Ethics for Nurses and Midwives*. London: NMC.

Nordenfelt, L. 2003. Dignity of elderly: An introduction. *Medicine, Health Care and Philosophy* 6(2): 99–101.

Patients Association. 2009. *Patients ... Not Numbers, People ... Not Statistics*. London: Patients Association.

Reed, P. 2011. Dignity for children. In Matiti, M.R., and Baillie, L. (eds.), *Dignity in Health Care for Nurses and Midwives: A Practical Approach for Nurses and Midwives*. London: Radcliffe, 81–94.

Royal College of Nursing (RCN). 2008. *Defending Dignity—Challenges and Opportunities*. London: RCN.

Royal College of Nursing (RCN). 2010. *Dignity in Health Care for People with Learning Disabilities—RCN Guidance*. London: RCN.

Royal College of Physicians. 2012. *Hospitals on the Edge? The Time for Action. A Report by the Royal College of Physicians*. Available from: http://www.rcplondon.ac.uk/sites/default/files/documents/hospitals-on-the-edge-report.pdf (accessed 22 June 2013).

Royal College of Psychiatrists. 2013. *Whole-Person Care: From Rhetoric to Reality. Achieving Parity between Mental and Physical Health*. Occasional paper OP88. http://www.rcpsych.ac.uk/files/pdfversion/OP88xx.pdf (accessed 22 April 2014).

Slettebø, A., Caspari, S., Lohne, V., Aasgaard, T., Nåden, D. 2009. Dignity in the life of people with head injuries. *Journal of Advanced Nursing* 65: 2426–2433.

Stacey, G., Stickley, T. 2011. Dignity in mental health: Listening to the flying saint. In Matiti, M., and Baillie, L. (eds.), *Dignity in Healthcare: A Practical Approach for Nurses and Midwives*. London: Radcliffe, 171–185.

Tadd, W., Bayer, T., Dieppe, P. 2002. Dignity in health care: Reality or rhetoric. *Reviews in Clinical Gerontology* 12(1): 1–4.

Thomas, S.A., Lee-Fong, M. 2010. Maintaining dignity of patients with morbid obesity in the hospital setting. *Bariatric Times* 8(4): 20–25.

Touhy, T.A., Brown, C., Smith, C.J. 2005. Spiritual caring: End of life in a nursing home. *Journal of Gerontological Nursing* 31(9): 27–35.

Valentine, N., Darby, C., Bonsel, G.J. 2008. Which aspects of quality of care are most important? Results from WHO's general population surveys of 'health system responsiveness' in 41 countries. *Social Science and Medicine* 66: 1939–1950.

Vohra, A.J.U., Brazil, K., Hanna, S., Abelson, J. 2004. Family perceptions of end-of-life care in long-term facilities. *Journal of Palliative Care* 20(4): 297–302.

Widäng, I., Fridlund, B. 2003. Self-respect, dignity and confidence: Conceptions of integrity among male patients. *Journal of Advanced Nursing* 42(1): 47–56.

Woogara, J. 2004. Patient privacy: An ethnographic study of privacy in NHS patient settings. Unpublished PhD thesis. University of Surrey.

Woolhead, G., Calnan, M., Dieppe, P., Tadd, W. 2005. Dignity in older age: What do older people in the United Kingdom think? *Age and Ageing* 33(2): 165–170.

World Health Organisation. 1994. *Declaration on the Promotion of Patients' Rights in Europe–Amsterdam*. Copenhagen: World Health Organisation Office for Europe.

7

Person-centred and holistic nursing care

Introduction

Person-centred approaches to health care are commonly advocated internationally (Cox 2011) and in the United Kingdom (UK), and the expectation to deliver care that is person centred and holistic is established in both professional and National Health Service (NHS) guidance. This chapter therefore explores the meaning of person-centred and holistic nursing care: working with people in a way that values and respects them as individuals, taking account of their individual needs, preferences and culture. We consider various models of care, with particular focus on areas of practice that have embraced person-centred care. We advise you to follow up with more specific reading on person-centred care in your field of practice.

Learning outcomes

By the end of this chapter, you will be able to

- Discuss the meaning of person-centred and holistic care, with reference to theories and models of care;
- Analyse the practices that promote person-centred and holistic care in different settings;
- Reflect on your own practice and experience in relation to person-centred care.

Background to person-centred care

Professional guidance and UK health policy set out the expectation for care delivery to be person centred and holistic. The Nursing and Midwifery Council (NMC) (2010) stated in the 'professional values' domain that nurses must be able to deliver person-centred nursing (PCN) care.

The NMC's (2008) Code also requires nurses to deliver care in a person-centred way:

> *You must treat people as individuals. You must listen to the people in your care and respond to their concerns and preferences.*
>
> *(p. 3)*

From a health policy perspective, the white paper *Liberating the NHS: Equity and Excellence* (Department of Health [DH] 2010), which laid the foundations for England's NHS reforms, included the principle of shared decision-making and 'no decision about me without me'. The NHS Constitution (DH 2013) set out that NHS services should

> *be coordinated around and tailored to, the needs and preferences of patients, their families and their carers. (p. 3) [...] We value every person—whether patient, their families or carers, or staff—as an individual, respect their aspirations and commitments in life, and seek to understand their priorities, needs, abilities and limits. (p. 5)*

Other UK countries have similar commitments to person-centred care. The Scottish government's (2010) healthcare strategy document aspires to consistent person-centred encounters for every person accessing health care and the provision of services that respect individual needs and values. Thus, the support for person-centred care in UK health policy appears unequivocal.

Although the focus in this chapter is on person-centred care, there are other related concepts used and discussed within healthcare literature. For example, 'patient-centred' care is the preferred term in America, using a definition developed by the Institute of Medicine (Patterson et al. 2011). Goodrich and Cornwell (2008) suggested that the phrase 'seeing the person in the patient' is most applicable to staff working in clinical practice. They further noted that the term *person-centred* care has been particularly used in the nursing and social work literature, and professions working with children more often use the term *family-centred* care; *relationship-centred* care is often used in care homes. Each of these alternatives is considered in this chapter.

The next section explores what we mean by 'person' and 'personhood'.

An exploration of person and personhood

In Chapter 1, we explored the nature of values, and we referred to the need to value each person in our care. The concepts of person and personhood are central to both caring and person-centredness (McCance et al. 2008).

Kitwood (1997), whose seminal work focussed on person-centred care for people with dementia, highlighted the uniqueness of each person and defined personhood as

> *a standing or status that is bestowed upon one human being, by others, in the context of relationship and social being. It implies recognition, respect and trust.* (p. 8)

In Chapter 6, in our analysis of the meaning of dignity, we considered the notion of human dignity that all human beings have. In 1948, after the atrocities of World War II were revealed and it was clear that many people had not been treated as human beings with dignity and rights, the United Nations published the Universal Declaration of Human Rights (UDHR). The UDHR is generally agreed to be the foundation of international human rights law, recognising the basic rights and fundamental freedoms inherent to all human beings and equally applicable to everyone, and that we are all born free and equal in dignity and rights.

Activity

Consider:

- What are the attributes of a human being—a person?
- Can you think of any examples when people accessing health care have not been treated as human beings?

McCormack (2004) explored the word *person* from a philosophical perspective, pointing out that although it is possible to see a person as a set of physical and psychological characteristics, such a viewpoint can lead to an individual not being treated as a person and instead being 'reduced to a "thing"' (p. 32). McCance et al. (2008) argued that the word *person* captures those attributes that represent our humanness and the factors that we regard as the most important and most challenging in our lives. Reports that have revealed poor-quality health care often refer to patients not being treated as people but as numbers. Indeed, a 2009 Patients Association report was titled 'Patients ... Not Numbers, People ... Not Statistics' and presented detailed case studies of poor care experiences. It is not unusual to hear staff referring to patients according to the patient's health condition or bed number, for example, 'the stroke in bed 18'. Staff who refer to patients in this way may nevertheless treat them as individual people, but there is a risk that thinking of and referring to patients as numbers or conditions will lead to care that is not person centred. For example, in Goodrich and Cornwell's (2008) study, patients described that they were moved about the hospital like 'a parcel'.

Ruddick (2010) suggested that the tendency to apply medical labels to mental health service users is counter to person-centredness, as labels mark the person as different and the label then directs future treatment. McCleod and McPherson (2007) reported that traditional approaches to medicine and health care focussed on treating the illness, according to its expected pattern, rather than considering each person as a unique individual. Health services are mainly organised according to medical diagnosis, for example, specialised units for people with certain conditions (e.g. the development of hyper-acute stroke units) or care pathways for people with particular diagnoses (e.g. fractured neck of femur). However, we must nevertheless focus on seeing the person in the unit or on a particular pathway as an individual. Goodrich and Cornwell (2008) investigated adult patients' experiences in acute hospitals, and all the patients and relatives they interviewed expressed the importance of being 'seen as a person' (p. 9), with their individual needs addressed, and being called by the name they preferred.

Person-centred care

The term *person-centred care* is increasingly used within the healthcare literature, but definitive definitions are more elusive. Nolan et al. (2004) commented that person-centred care is 'oft quoted but ill-defined' (p. 46), but they acknowledged that the concept has had considerable influence on policy, practice and academic literature, particularly in nursing. Similarly, McCance et al. (2008) stated that there is no one accepted definition of person-centredness, despite an increasing emphasis on the provision of person-centred care within healthcare systems.

Activity

Reflect on the term *person-centred care:*

- What do you think it might mean?
- If care is not person centred, what would it be like?
- Reflect on your care experiences: Can you identify any examples of when you feel that you or a colleague used a person-centred approach to care?

From the background provided previously in this chapter, you may have noticed that person-centred care is often linked with involvement in decision-making and addressing individual needs. McCance et al. (2008) suggested that person-centred care is broadly interpreted as treating people as individuals. The NMC (2010) defined person-centred nursing, as

> *care tailored to the individual needs and choices of the service user, taking into account diversity, culture, religion, spirituality, sexuality, gender, age, and disability.*
>
> *(p. 149)*

This definition implies a holistic approach, with care that addresses the individual person's diversity and preferences. In the previous activity, you might have remembered an example of where you discovered and addressed what mattered to a person in your care. This could be something as simple as enabling a person to make a telephone call that was important to the person. In a poignant example, Gallagher (2012) related how a student nurse went out to obtain an ice cream for a patient who was dying and desired a particular ice cream. Baillie (2014) gave the example of an intensive care nurse bringing in port and brandy from home, at the request of a man who was dying, and dipping mouth care sticks into the drink for him to taste. These practice examples of being person centred are clearly underpinned by values such as compassion and commitment. The Health Foundation (2013) asserted that in person-centred care, patients are viewed as equal partners in assessing, planning and developing care to ensure that it is appropriate. The foundation further suggested that core components of person-centred care are compassion, dignity and respect; shared decision-making; and collective patient and public involvement in service design and delivery.

Manley et al. (2011) suggested that person-centred care is recognised through a focus on getting to know the patient as a person (the person's values, beliefs, health and social care needs and preferences); enabling the patient to make decisions based on informed choices (through provision of individualised and evidence-based information); using shared decision-making between patients and healthcare teams; enabling choice of specific care and services to meet the patient's health and social care needs and preferences; providing ongoing evaluation of services for appropriateness with feedback from service users; and supporting the person to assert his or her choices.

Models of nursing

Traditionally, the nursing profession followed a medical model, focussing on the person's diagnosis, treatment and related care, but various nursing models of care, developed in the latter part of the twentieth century, countered this approach. Pearson et al. (2005) and

Fitzpatrick and Whall (2005) presented a range of nursing models, and all support holistic approaches to care that focus on the individual and are congruent with person-centred care approaches. Humanistic nursing theories, which focus on patients as human beings, particularly emphasise dignity, caring relationships, and the person as a holistic and unique individual (Watson 1988; Muetzel 1988; Orlando 1990). Schroeder (1992) claimed that all definitions of nursing make reference to a relationship between nurses and patients, implying that for nursing to take place there must be a relationship. Most nursing models originated in North America, but the Roper, Logan and Tierney model of care (Roper et al. 2000) was developed in the UK and remains widely used, often in an adapted form. This model addresses activities of daily living (ADLs) and considers each person's lifespan, independence, individuality in living, and factors (biological, psychological, sociocultural, and environmental and politicoeconomic) that influence how they carry out their ADLs. There have been criticisms that the model leads to a checklist approach to care and an over-emphasis on physical care needs (Ellis 1999). However, the application of any model of care is influenced by the underlying values of caregivers and the culture of the care environment.

Theories of person-centred care

In 2004, McCormack identified that although there is frequent reference to 'person-centred practice', systematic research into person-centred nursing practice was poorly developed. He reviewed the commonalities of various person-centred models, identifying core principles as knowing the person, values, biography, relationships, seeing beyond the immediate needs and authenticity. He argued that these models, although derived from differing practice perspectives, are all firmly rooted in a humanistic philosophical tradition. From a review of the literature at that time, McCormack (2004) suggested four concepts to underpin person-centred nursing: being in relation; being in a social world; being in place; being with self. Each of these is explored further next.

- *Being in relation*: Nurse-patient relationships are a core principle of person-centred care; many theories of nursing emphasise the nurse-patient relationship as central to caring and nursing practice (e.g. Peplau 1988; Watson 1988). McCance et al. (2008) considered that effective person-centred nursing requires the formation of therapeutic relationships, built on trust and understanding, between professionals, patients and others significant to them in their lives.

- *Being in a social world*: This concept recognises that people are social beings. Accordingly, narratives and biography are increasingly used in care of older people and particularly those with dementia.
- *Being in place:* This refers to the context in which care is provided and how the care environment affects each person and facilitation of person-centred care.
- *Being with self*: This concept relates to understanding what the person values in his or her life and helping the person to find meaning in personal care.

McCormack et al. (2008) proposed that principles of person-centeredness include respect for persons; the rights of individuals as persons; the values and beliefs of individuals; mutual respect and understanding; and the development of therapeutic relationships. McCormack and McCance (2010) developed the person-centred nursing framework, which is presented in detail in their textbook, *Person-Centred Nursing: Theory and Practice*. The framework has four constructs: pre-requisites (the attributes of the nurse, e.g. professional competence); the care environment (the context for care delivery, including systems and staffing); person-centred processes (how person-centred nursing is delivered, e.g. shared decision-making, holistic care); and expected outcomes (e.g. involvement in care, satisfaction with care).

Nolan et al. (2004) argued for 'relational care' rather than person-centred care to be applied in older people's care. They presented the 'Senses Framework', which is based on the belief that all those involved in caring (the older person, family carers, and paid or voluntary carers) should experience relationships that promote a sense of

> - *security—to feel safe within relationships;*
> - *belonging—to feel 'part' of things;*
> - *continuity—to experience links and consistency;*
> - *purpose—to have a personally valuable goal or goals;*
> - *achievement—to make progress towards a desired goal or goals;*
> - *significance—to feel that 'you' matter.*
>
> *(p. 49)*

My Home Life is a UK-wide evidence-based project to improve quality of life in care homes. The principles adopted include the 'Senses Framework' for developing relationships (see http://myhomelife.org.uk/research/8-key-themes//).

McCormack (2004) has asserted that person-centred care is more inclusive than relational care as it includes relationships anyway. He argued that viewing the person within the person's context is essential.

Factors influencing delivery of person-centred care

There are a range of factors that can affect the delivery of person-centred care and we explore these next.

Activity

Consider your own field of practice and your practice experience:

- How do the concepts of person-centred care relate to these settings?
- What helps and what hinders you in being person centred?

You might have considered various influencing factors, but the care environment, including organisational culture, is particularly important. In Chapter 6, we examined the care environment in relation to promoting dignity. As person-centred care and dignity are closely linked, it is not surprising that the care environment is also an important dimension for person-centred care. Manley et al. (2011) argued that for person-centred care to achieve its full potential, the approach needs to be practised by the entire nursing team. This requires a shared philosophy and ways of working that prioritise person-centred behaviour, not only with patients and those who are important to them, but also within the team. In relation to dementia, Kirkley et al. (2011) argued for a shared culture at all levels of the organisation to ensure person-centred dementia care. They found that participants highlighted resource constraints and the knowledge, attitudes and personal qualities of staff as barriers to implementing person-centred care. Leadership style and the way that managers support and value staff were other important influences. Manley et al. (2011) argued that the well-being of staff and how they are supported also needs to be person centred as staff well-being positively affects the care environment for staff and patients.

In 2011, the Royal College of Psychiatrists (RCP) published an audit of dementia care in hospitals and revealed minimal evidence of person-centred approaches being used in hospital wards, with care generally task related and the environment non-dementia friendly and impersonal. Webster (2011), in relation to acute hospitals, stated that the routinised nature of many ward environments, shift patterns, high staff turnover and weak clinical leadership acted as barriers to person-centred care. McCormack (2004) argued that with the challenges of everyday practice, it is more realistic to strive for a constant state of becoming more person centred in our practice, rather than achieving an ideal of person-centredness. Edvardsson et al. (2010) identified that flexible routines adapted to residents' needs rather than staff needs promoted a person-centred approach. Baillie et al. (2012) gave several examples of where student nurses were creative and adapted ward routines for people with dementia in hospital.

McCormack (2004) highlighted that although person-centred care has often been applied to specific contexts (notably involving older people, particularly those with dementia), as a concept it is applicable much more generally. The application of person-centred care is now explored in relation to the care of older people and people with dementia, people with learning disabilities, mental health care settings, and care of children and families (family-centred care).

Person-centred care for older people and people with dementia

Much of the dialogue in the literature about person-centred care focusses on older people and particularly people with dementia. The DH (2001a) published the *National Service Framework for Older People*, which included a standard for 'person-centred care', and stated that person-centred care requires managers and professionals to listen to older people, respect their dignity and privacy, recognise individual differences and specific needs, enable older people to make informed choices, involve them in all decisions about their needs and care, provide coordinated and integrated service responses, and involve and support carers whenever necessary. Webster (2011) argued that the capacity of person-centred care to improve care suggests that it needs to be embedded in older people's nursing practice in acute hospital settings as a clinical and managerial priority.

Person-centred approaches to care are increasingly considered to be synonymous with best-quality care for people with dementia (Edvardsson et al. 2010). Kitwood's (1997) work on person-centred approaches for people with dementia (mentioned previously in this chapter) developed dementia care mapping (DCM), which is a process that attempts to help practitioners put themselves in the place of people with dementia when evaluating the quality of care. DCM is increasingly used for developing person-centred care for people with dementia, across general hospitals as well as in units dedicated to care of people with dementia. As another framework for person-centred care, Brooker (2004, 2007) recommended the VIPS framework: V for valuing people with dementia and carers, I for treating people as individuals, P for using the perspective of the person with dementia and S for a positive social environment. Edvardsson et al. (2010), in a study based in residential care, found that the core category of person-centred care was promoting a continuation of self and normality, which was achieved through knowing the person; welcoming family; providing meaningful activities; being in a personalised environment; and experiencing flexibility and continuity.

Activity

A hospital setting can be a frightening and disorientating place for anyone but particularly for a person with dementia.

- Reflect on what practices you have seen to promote normality for people with dementia.
- Consider: How could nurses promote normality in an outpatient environment, an emergency department or a hospital ward?

Edvardsson et al. (2010) provided various examples of promoting normality in residential care, but most of these could be adapted for any other setting. Suggestions include addressing the person in a way that acknowledges them as valuable and competent through finding out how the person likes to be addressed; providing opportunities to do things that the person enjoys (e.g. listening to music, looking at photographs); enabling the person to make decisions about when to eat or get up (some acute hospital wards have snacks readily available, and routines can often be adapted to enable choice); and spending time with family, through welcoming family and supporting flexible visiting, including overnight stays. In Edvardsson et al.'s (2010) study, all participants described that knowing the history, preferences, needs, interests and particular wishes of the person receiving care was fundamental for person-centred care. They further expressed that it was essential to apply this understanding in practice, through initiating conversations, activities and routines that were meaningful for the person.

You might also have considered how you could adapt the care environment, an aspect recognised as important in person-centred care frameworks. The King's Fund includes a number of resources to support staff to develop environments that are more supportive for people with dementia in hospitals and care homes (see http://www.kingsfund.org.uk/projects/enhancing-healing-environment/ehe-design-dementia). There are many good examples of adapting care settings for people with dementia. In Edvardsson et al.'s (2010) study, all participants referred to personalising the environment; an example was enriching the environment with personal things like photographs, furniture, plants, decorations and other memorabilia familiar to the person with dementia or that they were known to like. Personal things could contribute to person-centredness by supporting the identity and continuation of self for the person with dementia; by prompting meaningful conversation and providing areas for reminiscence; by enabling recognition and possibly feelings of being at home in the setting; and by reminding staff of the person's uniqueness. As an example in hospital, Sanders and Webster (2011) explained how, with charitable funding, a six-bed bay for people with dementia in a trauma ward was decorated and furnished to provide a homely atmosphere with a sense of calm. With families' input, personal care plans were introduced to enable staff to learn more about each person and to help them to communicate their likes, dislikes, needs and wants. Families were encouraged to bring in personal and familiar belongings for patients, and open visiting was introduced so that relatives could have greater involvement in care.

Biography

The use of biography, or life story work, is increasingly used for understanding individuals' perspectives. Life story work involves working with a person or the person's family to find out about the person's life and use this information with the person in their care (McKeown et al. 2006). McKeown et al. (2010) argued that life story work has the potential to enable care staff to see the person behind the patient; allow family carers to uphold their relatives' personhood; enable the voice of the person with dementia to be heard, verbally and non-verbally; be enjoyable for all concerned, and enable the person with dementia to feel proud about themselves and their lives. Clarke et al. (2003) argued that the biographical approach encourages nurses to discover the 'person behind the patient' and the individual's attitudes, aspirations, past experiences and life history. They found that use of photographs removed stereotypes and assumptions, prompted communication and therefore enhanced nurse-patient relationships.

Much of the published biographical literature has focussed on residential care (Russell and Timmons 2009; Edvardsson et al. 2010; Kellett et al. 2010). Although carrying out detailed life story work may not be feasible in hospital, staff can find out about important aspects of a person's life. As an example, students in Baillie et al.'s (2012) study discussed their strategies for getting to know older people with dementia, for example, engaging in conversation about the older person's life and talking to their families. One student described how a former naval captain kept packing his bags and attempting to leave the ward to 'go to sea'. The student engaged him in conversation about the navy: 'He started telling me about all the ports and places he'd been; what he had done during his service' (p. 23).

The Alzheimer's Society has produced a leaflet 'This Is Me', with spaces for photos and information, to support people with dementia, so that nurses and other healthcare staff can better understand the person's perspectives and take into account their preferences. When caring for people with dementia, be proactive about using 'This Is Me' (available from http://www.alzheimers.org.uk/site/scripts/documents_info.php?documentID=1290) and getting to know the person and the person's family. The RCP (2011) recommended that a personal information document, like 'This Is Me', should be implemented in hospitals. In Baillie et al.'s (2012) study, one student mentioned a similar document:

> *She came in with a beautiful book with pictures and words and the kind of things you could point at, so you could communicate with her. So it's more of a—similar to a passport, so it had information in there for communication and what she liked and what she didn't like.*
>
> (*p. 23*)

Such documents help staff get to know the person quickly, which assists with forming a relationship even in a short-stay environment. A caregiver who gets to know a person with dementia is better placed to initiate conversations and meaningful activities (Edvardsson et al. 2010).

Activity

If you have cared for a person with dementia in practice, consider:

- What did you know about the person and how did you know this? How could you have gotten to know the person better?
- What familiar personal belongings did the person have? Could you and others have done more to personalise the person's environment?

Person-centred approaches to care of people with learning disabilities

The DH (2001b) published *Valuing People: A New Strategy for Learning Disability for the 21st Century*, which stressed that people with learning disabilities are people first, and there should be a focus on what they can do rather than what they cannot. As a follow-up, the DH (2009) published *Valuing People Now: A New Three-Year Strategy for Learning Disabilities*, which acknowledged that access to the NHS is often poor and characterised by problems that undermine personalisation, dignity and safety. Carnaby et al. (2010) identified that *Valuing People Now* provides a clear central message: that all people with learning disabilities should have the same rights and choices as other citizens. The website Improving Health and Lives Observatory (http://www.improvinghealthandlives.org.uk/) monitors the health and health care of people with learning disabilities and includes a hospital Traffic Light Assessment that, when completed, gives hospital staff important information about a person with learning disabilities who is admitted to hospital (see http://www.improvinghealthandlives.org.uk/adjustments/?adjustment=70). In a review of deaths in hospital of people with learning disabilities, Heslop et al. (2013) reported that, despite evidence to suggest that a hospital 'passport' (a patient profile document or 'traffic light' document) helped nursing staff to understand a person's needs and provide person-centred nursing care, only a fifth (19%) of the patients reviewed had such a document. Now, review the scenario and questions in Box 7.1.

Box 7.1

Practice scenario: person-centred care

Sarah is 26 years old and has a moderate learning disability. Five years ago, she moved into her own flat, where she is supported by a key worker, Naomi, who is also her 'health facilitator'. Sarah likes listening to music and attends activities at a day centre, where she enjoys socialising with other people. Sarah has infrequent contact with her parents, who are divorced, and rarely sees her sisters, but she has regular contact with an aunt. Sarah can communicate verbally, but her speech impediment means that people who do not know her often have difficulty understanding her at first. Sarah has asthma and attends her practice nurse's clinic, accompanied by Naomi, to monitor her condition. Unfortunately, twice in the last year, Sarah developed severe wheezing and attended the emergency department, on one occasion staying overnight. She found the experience distressing, particularly as she had to have blood taken.

Questions

1. Access the hospital Traffic Light Assessment document (http://www.improvinghealthandlives.org.uk/adjustments/?adjustment=70). How might Sarah taking a completed document like this to future health appointments help promote person-centred care for her?
2. How could a community learning disability nurse work with Sarah, Naomi and the practice nurse to better support person-centred care for Sarah?

Camble (2012) asserted that staff must avoid labelling of people with learning disabilities and that diagnostic overshadowing can occur, with all aspects of clients' behaviours seen to be caused by their learning disabilities and therefore 'normal'. Clearly, such approaches run counter to person-centred care, but there are reports of the underlying causes of behaviour, such as anxiety or pain, being overlooked (Royal College of Nursing 2010), sometimes with serious consequences (Mencap 2012).

Various initiatives to improve person-centred care for people with learning disabilities have been reported. Camble (2012) explained how the approach of a charity (United Response) uses 'person-centred active support' for working with clients in the community, providing care that is 'done with' rather than 'done to' service users and highlighting the need to get to know them as individuals and look beyond their reputation, diagnosis or label. In a further example, Carnaby et al. (2010) reported on a flexible response service model, which took a person-centred approach to meeting needs, with social inclusion and citizenship at the core. They provided varying support–assessment, short-term and long-term interventions–for people with learning disabilities, with a focus on providing a 'capable' environment to support people with multiple needs, for example, when people have serious physical illness and need support with treatments, including renal dialysis and invasive investigations.

Person-centred care in mental health

In an influential review of mental health nursing, the chief nursing officer for England asserted the following:

> *Developing and sustaining positive therapeutic relationships with service users, their families and/or carers should form the basis of all care.*
>
> *(DH 2006, p. 4)*

Shattel et al. (2007) asserted that clients want nurses to take the time to know them as a whole person, rather than as a service user. Ruddick (2010) explained that within mental health care, person-centred approaches draw on the work of Carl Rogers (1951) and the belief that humans flourish through therapeutic relationships, which rely on core conditions: acceptance, genuineness and empathic understanding. Such an approach requires a non-judgemental attitude and 'unconditional positive regard' to provide a safe environment for people to explore their most sensitive thoughts and feelings (Ruddick 2010). Ruddick (2010) further argued that true person-centred care follows from genuine engagement with the person who is disclosing personal fears and aspirations.

Stacey and Stickley (2011) explained that recovery has centre place in contemporary mental health policy. Ruddick (2010) argued that the recovery model requires a person-centred approach to enable service users to 'explore their thoughts and feelings, re-author their lives and discover a more accepting sense of self' (p. 24). In 2011, the National Institute for Health and Clinical Excellence (NICE) published best practice advice for improving the experience of people who use adult NHS mental health services. The guidance intent is to promote person-centred care, taking into account people's needs, preferences and strengths. Spending time 'being with' a client reinforces the fact that the client is valued, irrespective of any therapeutic strategies that might follow (Ruddick 2010). However, person-centred care can be constrained by task-oriented systems and pressured work, with more importance placed on targets than on the quality of nurse-client interactions (Ruddick 2010).

As an example of person-centred care in practice, Oldknow et al. (2012) explained care pathways in a unit where staff offer health and social support and devise pathways of care for people with significant mental illness or challenging behaviour and coexisting physical illness. The work includes intensive person-centred work with the individuals concerned, and their families, carers and advocates, to achieve agreed recovery goals. Oldknow et al. (2012) argued that person-centred plans can decrease the risk, frequency, duration and intensity of challenging behaviour.

Family-centred care

Family-centred care models are considered to be a central tenet of children's nursing (Corlett and Twycross 2006) and the best way to provide care to children in hospital (Shields et al. 2012). Shields et al. (2006) defined family-centred care as

> *a way of caring for children and their families within health services which ensures that care is planned around the whole family, not just the individual child/person, and in which all the family members are recognized as care recipients.*
>
> *(p. 1318)*

Family-centred care approaches acknowledge that when a child is admitted, the whole family is affected, so staff must consider the impact of the child's admission on the whole family (Shields et al. 2012). In a review of qualitative studies, Shields et al. (2006) identified that effective negotiation between staff and families was essential for family-centred care, along with clarifying the roles of staff and families in the child's care. A number of studies have focussed on family-centred care in particular settings, for example, neonatal care (Staniszewska et al. 2012; Trajkovski et al. 2012). The studies all highlighted that getting to know the families, partnership and involvement are central to family-centred care. In a survey of children's nurses across Ireland, respondents perceived family-centred care to include family involvement, working in partnership, negotiating care, delivery of high-quality care and a multi-disciplinary approach (Coyne et al. 2011). Smith et al. (2010) presented a practice continuum for family-centred care, with varying levels of family involvement across the continuum, and including scenarios illustrating application.

From a systematic review of studies evaluating family-centred care, Shields et al. (2012) identified some benefits for children's clinical care, parental satisfaction, and costs. Coyne et al. (2011) found that although nurses accepted family-centred care as an ideal philosophy for the care of children and their families, the implementation of family-centred care in practice posed some challenges for nurses, who indicated that they required further organisational and managerial support to fully implement family-centred care practices. From a review of the literature, Corlett and Twycross (2006) revealed that the essential negotiation processes involved were not routinely planned or conducted and that 'the reality in practice does not match the rhetoric' (p. 1315). They recommended that for family-centred care to be a reality, nurses need to communicate with children and their families effectively so that parents can negotiate their participation in care with health staff and be involved in the decision-making process. Thus, to summarise, although family-centred care is well established in children's nursing, it appears that application in practice still needs refining. Smith and Coleman's (2010) text reviewed child- and family-centred health care in detail in the context of health and social policy and is useful further reading.

Family-centred care in adult nursing

In adult care, the term *family-centred care* is used infrequently, although involvement of family is included in person-centred care frameworks, implicitly if not explicitly. There are few reports of family-centred care for adults in the literature, and those available tend to focus on visiting hours in hospital (e.g. Soury-Lavergne et al. 2011).

Activity

Reflect on any experiences you have in adult care settings and to what extent care is family centred. Consider:

- How do the staff work with, and involve, families?
- What are the visiting hours? If they are restricted, reflect on the impact of these restrictions on patients and their families.
- How are families involved? Could they be more involved? How might this affect patients' and their families' experiences?
- If you have been in hospital as an adult, or had an adult family member in hospital, reflect on your personal experience of family involvement.

Holistic and person-centred care

The concept of holistic care in nursing emerged to combat the 'medical model of care', whereby people were cared for solely according to their medical diagnosis.

Read the case study in Box 7.2 and consider the questions posed.

Box 7.2

Practice scenario: holistic and person-centred care

Martin is 53 years old and divorced and lives alone in a housing association flat. Martin's mother recently died, and he has been having difficulty coming to terms with his loss. Martin does some part-time work but has been unable to work recently and is worried about paying his bills. Martin has a long-standing diagnosis of schizophrenia and is under the care of the community mental health team. One Sunday, Martin visited the emergency department after an episode of chest pain. After an initial assessment, he was admitted to the medical admissions unit for monitoring. After 2 days, he was discharged, with an appointment for the cardiology outpatient division. He was also advised that he should make an appointment with the practice nurse for blood pressure monitoring as he was hypertensive. His community mental health team was informed of his admission.

Questions

- What factors might affect Martin's health and well-being and how might these inter-relate?
- How can nurses and other healthcare professionals work together using a person-centred approach to promote holistic care for Martin?

The RCP (2013) noted the close relationship between mental health and physical health and that this influence works in both directions as poor mental health is associated with a greater risk of physical health problems, and poor physical health is associated with a greater risk of mental health problems. If Martin's care in the acute hospital focussed solely on his physical symptoms and the associated medical diagnosis, such an approach would not meet his individual needs in a holistic way. The social factors included in the scenario will also have a major impact on his physical and mental health. The RCP (2013) emphasised that in holistic care, the mind and the body should not be regarded separately but integrated.

Byatt (2008) asserted that holistic care is an approach or value system held by practitioners who provide care which recognises the patient as a whole person with physical, psychological, sociological and spiritual dimensions. A concept analysis of the term *holistic nursing practice* led to the following working definition for application by nurses in practice:

> *Holistic nursing care embraces the mind, body and spirit of the patient, in a culture that supports a therapeutic nurse/patient relationship, resulting in wholeness, harmony and healing. Holistic care is patient led and patient focused in order to provide individualised care, thereby, caring for the patient as a whole person rather than in fragmented parts.*
>
> *(McEvoy and Duffy 2008, p. 418)*

The definition emphasises patients as individuals and as a whole and highlights the importance of nurse-patient relationships–a central tenet in person-centred care. You will also see that the definition of holistic care refers to 'mind, body, and spirit', a concept often referred to in sources exploring holistic practice. Cox (2011) argued that the biopsychosocial model of care was conceived as a scientific, rather than a values, framework that would hold together the biological and psychological sciences. Cox suggested that a body-mind-spirit model, which includes meaning and purpose as well as spirituality, is useful for considering the complexity of person-centred care.

Miner-Williams (2006) suggested that spirituality is the essence of being human and can include meaning and connectedness as well as important values and beliefs. There is growing evidence for links between spirituality and human health, healing and well-being (Sessanna et al. 2007; Koslander et al. 2009). However, Koslander et al. (2009) highlighted that even though people with mental health problems often have spiritual care needs, these have not always been addressed. Miner-Williams (2006) suggested that a meaningful assessment of spirituality includes asking questions such as 'How are your spirits today?' or 'How does being in hospital affect you and your family?' and, most important, shows a genuine interest in the person.

Culture

The United Kingdom is an increasingly diverse society, and all care must be carried out with sensitivity and in a culturally appropriate manner for each individual and family. The American nurse and anthropologist Madeleine Leininger studied transcultural caring over many years and identified how acts of caring such as comforting and physical care, and the meaning attached to them, can vary between cultures (Leininger 1981). Leininger suggested that culture and caring cannot be separated within nursing actions and decision-making. Papadopoulos (2006a) presented the Papadopoulos–Tilki–Taylor model for transcultural nursing and health, consisting of four linked elements: cultural awareness, cultural knowledge, cultural sensitivity and cultural competence.

Cultural awareness includes examining and questioning your personal value base and beliefs. Chapter 1 of this book helped you explore your values.

Cultural knowledge may be drawn from sources such as sociology, anthropology and research, but you can learn a great deal about different cultures through experience with people. Learning about cultural and religious practices before and after death is important, but there will always be individual variations and needs. A person-centred approach requires you to build a relationship with the individual person you are caring for and the person's family and find out what their wishes are as you must avoid stereotyping. Leever (2011) reported on examples of nurses taking time to listen to patients so they could understand the patients' perspectives and were able to adjust care delivery so that it was culturally comfortable and acceptable.

Cultural sensitivity can be achieved by nurses working with people as partners, offering choices in care (see Chapter 8, "Working in Partnership"). In Cioffi's (2005) study, when caring for culturally diverse patients, one nurse said: 'If I am not sure, I just say to the patient "What is the right thing for me to do?", "Can I do this" or "Would you mind if I do this?"' Another nurse said: 'It's just finding out what they believe and what they don't believe in and then you can work it out from there with them and individualise their care.' Communication skills, respect and empathy are all important for cultural sensitivity.

Cultural competence requires the application of cultural awareness, knowledge and sensitivity to achieve effective health care that addresses people's cultural beliefs, behaviour and needs. A culturally competent nurse also challenges prejudice, discrimination and inequality (see Chapter 1 for an exploration of anti-discriminatory practice). Leishman (2006) highlighted the importance of mental health nurses developing cultural competence in an increasingly culturally diverse UK society.

Activity

Reflect on your own cultural competence and jot down a few notes about

- your personal values and beliefs,
- your cultural knowledge, and
- your skills that will help you to demonstrate cultural sensitivity.

Chapter summary

Person-centred and holistic approaches to care are well established in health policy and professional guidance and are closely aligned to humanistic nursing theories and models. A range of theories that underpin person-centred care exists; some of these were developed within specific care contexts. Core principles of all these approaches are to recognise the value of people as human beings and their personhood and to value each person's uniqueness as an individual. Developing a relationship with the person and the person's family, and learning about their life and what matters to them, is essential for person-centred care, as is seeing the person as a whole rather than focussing on their dominant health condition. In children's nursing, family-centred care is well established and accepted, but in person-centred care for adults, family involvement is also integral. Person-centred care is a vast topic, and there are many useful texts focussing in depth on person-centred care applied to particular contexts, for example, for people with dementia or people with learning disabilities. An important aspect of person-centred care in any setting is partnership, and this is considered in more depth in Chapter 8.

References

Baillie, L. 2014. Practical nursing skills: A caring approach. In Baillie, L. (ed.), *Developing Practical Adult Nursing Skills,* 4th ed. Boca Raton, FL: Taylor & Francis, 1–31.

Baillie, L., Merritt, J., Cox, J. 2012. Caring for older people with dementia in hospital: Part two: Strategies. *Nursing Older People* 24(9): 22–26.

Brooker, D. 2004. What is person-centred care in dementia? *Reviews in Clinical Gerontology* 13: 215–222.

Brooker, D. 2007. *Person Centred Dementia Care: Making Services Better.* London: Kingsley.

Byatt, K. 2008. Holistic care. In Mason-Whitehead, E., Mcintosh, A., Bryan, A., and Mason, T. (eds.), *Key Concepts in Nursing.* Los Angeles: Sage, 168–174.

Camble, A. 2012. Person-centred support of people who exhibit challenging behaviour. *Learning Disability in Practice* 15(2): 18–20.

Carnaby, S., Roberts, B., Lang, J., Nielsen, P. 2010. A flexible response: Person-centred support and social inclusion for people with learning disabilities and challenging behaviour. *British Journal of Learning Disabilities* 39: 39–45.

Cioffi, J. 2005. Nurses' experiences of caring for culturally diverse patients in an acute care setting. *Contemporary Nurse* 20(1): 78–96.

Clarke, A., Hanson, E., Ross, H. 2003. Seeing the person behind the patient: Enhancing the care of older people using a biographical approach. *Journal of Clinical Nursing* 12(5): 697–706.

Corlett, J., Twycross, A. 2006. Negotiation of parental roles within family-centred care: A review of the research. *Journal of Clinical Nursing* 15(10): 1308–1316.

Cox, J.L. 2011. Empathy, identity and engagement in person-centred medicine: The sociocultural context. *Journal of Evaluation in Clinical Practice* 17: 350–353.

Coyne, I., O'Neill, C., Murphy, M., Costello, T., O'Shea, R. 2011. What does family-centred care mean to nurses and how do they think it could be enhanced in practice. *Journal of Advanced Nursing* 67(12): 2561–2573.

Department of Health (DH). 2001a. *National Service Framework for Older People*. London: DH.

Department of Health (DH). 2001b. *Valuing People: A New Strategy for Learning Disability for the 21st Century*. London: DH.

Department of Health (DH). 2006. *From Values to Actions: The Chief Nursing Officer's Review of Mental Health Nursing*. London: DH.

Department of Health (DH). 2009. *Valuing People Now: A New Three-Year Strategy for Learning Disabilities*. London: DH.

Department of Health (DH). 2010. *Liberating the NHS: Equity and Excellence*. London: DH.

Department of Health (DH). 2013. *The NHS Constitution for England*. Available from: https://www.gov.uk/government/publications/the-nhs-constitution-for-england (accessed 24 November 2013).

Edvardsson, D., Fetherstonhaugh, D., Nay, R. 2010. Promoting a continuation of self and normality: Person-centred care as described by people with dementia, their family members and aged care staff. *Journal of Clinical Nursing* 19: 2611–2618.

Ellis, S. 1999. The patient-centred care model: Holistic multiprofessional/reflective. *British Journal of Nursing* 8: 5, 296–301.

Fitzpatrick, J.J., Whall, A.L. 2005. *Conceptual Models of Nursing: Analysis and Application*. Englewood Cliffs, NJ: Prentice Hall.

Gallagher, A. 2012. Acknowledging small acts of kindness. *Nursing Ethics* 19(3): 311–312.

Goodrich, J., Cornwell, J. 2008. *Seeing the Person in the Patient: The Point of Care Review Paper.* London: King's Fund.

Health Foundation. 2013. *Person-Centred Care*. Available from: http://www.health.org.uk/areas-of-work/topics/person-centred-care/person-centred-care/ (accessed 1 October 2013).

Heslop, P., Blair, P., Fleming, P., Hoghton, M., Marriott, A., Russ, L. 2013. *Confidential Inquiry into Premature Deaths of People with Learning Disabilities.* Available from: http://www.bris.ac.uk/cipold/fullfinalreport.pdf (accessed 10 October 2013).

Kellett, U., Moyle, W., McAllister, M., et al. 2010. Life stories and biography: A means of connecting family and staff to people with dementia. *Journal of Clinical Nursing* 19(11–12): 1707–1715.

Kirkley, C., Bamford, C., Poole, M., Arksey, H., Hughes, J., Bond, J. 2011. The impact of organisational culture on the delivery of person-centred care in services providing respite care and short breaks for people with dementia. *Health & Social Care in the Community* 19(4): 438–448.

Kitwood, T. 1997. *Dementia Reconsidered: The Person Comes First.* Buckingham, UK: Open University Press.

Koslander, T., da Silva, A.B., Roxberg, A. 2009. Existential and spiritual needs in mental health care: An ethical and holistic perspective. *Journal of Holistic Nursing* 27: 34–42.

Leever, M.G. 2011. Cultural competence: Reflections on patient autonomy and patient good. *Nursing Ethics* 18(4): 560–557.

Leininger, M. 1981. Transcultural nursing: Its progress and its future. *Nursing and Health Care* 2: 365–371.

Leishman, J.L. 2006. Culturally sensitive mental health care: A module for 21st century education and practice. *International Journal of Psychiatric Nursing Research* 11(3): 1310–1321.

Manley, K, Hills, V., Marriot, S. 2011. Person-centred care: Principles of nursing practice D. *Nursing Standard* 25(31): 35–37.

McCance, T., Slater, P., McCormack, B. 2008. Using the caring dimensions inventory as an indicator of person-centred nursing. *Journal of Clinical Nursing* 18: 409–417.

McCleod, R., McPherson, K.M. 2007. Care and compassion: Part of person-centred rehabilitation, inappropriate response or a forgotten art? *Disability and Rehabilitation* 29(20–21): 1589–1595.

McCormack, B. 2004. Person-centredness in gerontological nursing: An overview of the literature. *International Journal of Older People Nursing in association with the Journal of Clinical Nursing* 13: 31–38.

McCormack, B., McCance, T. 2010. *Person-Centred Nursing: Theory and Practice.* Chichester, UK: Wiley Blackwell.

McCormack, B., McCance, T., Slater, P., McCormick, J., McArdle, C., Dewing, J. 2008. Person-centred outcomes and cultural change. In Manley, K., McCormack, B., Wilson, V. (eds.), *International Practice Development in Nursing and Healthcare.* Oxford, UK: Blackwell, 189–214.

McEvoy, L., Duffy, A. 2008. Holistic practice–a concept analysis. *Nurse Education in Practice* 8: 412–419.

McKeown, J., Clarke, A., Ingleton, C., Ryan, T., Repper, J. 2010. The use of life story work with people with dementia to enhance person-centred care. *International Journal of Older People Nursing* 5: 148–158.

McKeown, J., Clarke, A., Repper, J. 2006. Life story work in health and social care: Systematic literature review. *Journal of Advanced Nursing* 55: 237–247.

Mencap. 2012. *Death by Indifference: 74 Deaths and Counting: A Progress Report 5 Years On*. London: Mencap.

Miner-Williams, D. 2006. Putting a puzzle together: Making spirituality meaningful for nursing using an evolving theoretical framework. *Journal of Clinical Nursing* 15: 811–821.

Muetzel, P.A. 1988. Therapeutic nursing. In Pearson, A. (ed.), *Primary Nursing: Nursing in Burford and Oxford Nursing Development Units*. London: Chapman & Hall, 89–116.

National Institute for Health and Clinical Excellence. 2011. *Service User Experience in Adult Mental Health: Improving the Experience of Care for People Using Adult NHS Mental Health Services.* Clinical Guideline 136. Available from: http://publications.nice.org.uk/service-user-experience-in-adult-mental-health-improving-the-experience-of-care-for-people-using-cg136/person-centred-care (accessed 1 November 2013).

Nolan, M.R., Davies, S., Brown, J., Keady, J., Nolan, J. 2004. Beyond 'person-centred' care: A new vision for gerontological nursing. *International Journal of Older People Nursing in association with Journal of Clinical Nursing* 13, 3a: 45–53.

Nursing and Midwifery Council (NMC). 2008. *The Code: Standards of Conduct, Performance and Ethics for Nurses and Midwives.* London: NMC.

Nursing and Midwifery Council (NMC). 2010. *Standards for Pre-registration Nursing Education*. London: NMC.

Oldknow, H., Cornish, A., Newman, D. 2012. Communication and collaboration in person-centred care planning. *Learning Disability in Practice* 15(3): 19–22.

Orlando, I.J. 1990. *The Dynamic Nurse–Patient Relationship*. New York: National League for Nursing.

Papadopoulos, I. 2006a. The Papadopoulos, Tilki and Taylor model of developing cultural competence. In Papadopoulos, I. (ed.), *Transcultural Health and Social Care: Development of Culturally Competent Practitioners.* Edinburgh: Churchill Livingstone, 7–24.

Patients Association. 2009. *Patients ... Not Numbers, People ... Not Statistics.* London: Patients Association.

Patterson, M., Nolan, M., Rick, J., Brown, J., Adams, R., Musson, G. 2011. *From Metrics to Meaning: Culture Change and Quality of Acute Hospital Care for Older People: Report for the National Institute for Health Research Service Delivery and Organisation Programme*. Available from: http://www.ipfcc.org/resources/guidance/index.html (accessed 1 November 2013).

Pearson, A., Vaughan, B., Fitzgerald, M. 2005. *Nursing Models for Practice*. 3rd ed. Edinburgh: Butterworth Heinemann.

Peplau, H.E. 1988. *Interpersonal Relations in Nursing*. Hampshire, UK: Macmillan Education.

Rogers, C.R. 1951. *Client-Centered Therapy: Its Current Practices, Implications and Theory*. Boston: Houghton Mifflin.

Roper, N., Logan, W.W., Tierney, A.J. 2000. *The Roper-Logan-Tierney Model of Nursing: Based on Activities of Living*. Oxford, UK: Elsevier Health Sciences.

Royal College of Nursing. 2010. *Dignity in Healthcare for People with Learning Disabilities—RCN Guidance*. London: Royal College of Nursing.

Royal College of Psychiatrists (RCP). 2011. *Report of the National Audit of Dementia Care in General Hospitals*. Young, J., Hood, C., Woolley, R., Gandesha, A., Souza, R. (eds.). London: Healthcare Quality Improvement Partnership.

Royal College of Psychiatrists (RCP). 2013. *Whole-Person Care: From Rhetoric to Reality. Achieving Parity between Mental and Physical Health*. Occasional paper OP88. London: RCP.

Ruddick, F. 2010. Person-centred mental health care: Myth or reality? *Mental Health Practice* 13(9): 24–28.

Russell, C., Timmons, S. 2009. Life story work and nursing home residents with dementia. *Nursing Older People* 21(4): 28–32.

Sanders, K., Webster, J. 2011. Enabling dignity in care through practice development. In Matiti, M., and Baillie, L. (eds.), *Dignity in Healthcare: A Practical Approach for Nurses and Midwives*. London: Radcliffe, 220–238.

Schroeder, C. 1992. The process of inflicting pain in nursing: Caring relationship or torture. In Gaut, D.A. (ed.), *The Presence of Caring in Nursing*. New York: National League for Nursing, 211–220.

Scottish Government 2010. *The Healthcare Quality Strategy for NHS Scotland. Edinburgh*. Available from: http://www.scotland.gov.uk/Resource/Doc/311667/0098354.pdf (accessed 30 November 2013).

Sessanna, L., Finnell, D., Jezewski, M.A. 2007. Spirituality in nursing and health-related literature: A concept analysis. *Journal of Holistic Nursing* 25/4: 252–262.

Shattel, M., Starr, S., Thomas, P. 2007. 'Take my hand, help me out': Mental health service recipients' experience of the therapeutic relationship. *International Journal of Mental Health Nursing* 16: 274–284.

Shields, L., Pratt, J., Hunter, J. 2006. Family centred care: A review of qualitative studies. *Journal of Clinical Nursing* 15: 1317–1323.

Shields, L., Zhou, H., Pratt, J., Taylor, M., Hunter, J., Pascoe, E. 2012. Family-centred care for hospitalised children aged 0–12 years. *Cochrane Database of Systematic Reviews* 17: 10.

Smith, L., Coleman, V. 2010. *Child and Family-Centred Healthcare: Concept, Theory and Practice.* 2nd ed. Basingstoke, UK: Palgrave Macmillan.

Smith, L., Coleman, V., Bradshaw, M. 2010. Family-centred care: A practice continuum. In Smith, L., Coleman, V. (eds.), *Child and Family-Centred Healthcare: Concept, Theory and Practice.* 2nd ed. Basingstoke, UK: Palgrave Macmillan, 27–57.

Soury-Lavergne, A., Hauchard, I., Dray, S., et al. 2011. Survey of caregiver opinions on the practicalities of family-centred care in intensive care units. *Journal of Clinical Nursing* 21: 1060–1067.

Stacey, G., Stickley, T. 2011. Dignity in mental health: Listening to the flying saint. In Matiti, M., and Baillie, L. (eds.), *Dignity in Healthcare: A Practical Approach for Nurses and Midwives.* London: Radcliffe, 171–185.

Staniszewska, S., Brett, J., Redshaw, M., Hamilton, K., Newburn, M., Jones, N., Taylor, L. 2012. The POPPY study: Developing a model of family-centred care for neonatal units. *Worldviews on Evidence-Based Nursing* 9(4): 243–255.

Trajkovski, S., Schmied, V., Vickers, M., Jackson, D. 2012. Neonatal nurses' perspectives of family-centred care: A qualitative study. *Journal of Clinical Nursing* 21(17/18): 2477–2487.

United Nations. 1948. *Universal Declaration of Human Rights.* Available from: http://www.un.org/en/documents/udhr/ (accessed 1 October 2013).

Watson, J. 1988. *Nursing: Human Science and Human Care: A Theory of Nursing.* New York: National League for Nursing.

Webster, J. 2011. Improving care for people with dementia in acute hospital: The role of person-centred assessment. *Quality in Ageing & Older Adults* 12(2): 86–94.

8

Working in partnership with service users, carers and families

Introduction

Traditionally, health care was delivered using a paternalistic approach, with little active involvement from patients and families. However, health policy and guidelines for professionals now promote working in partnership with people accessing health care, with an expectation of shared decision-making about treatment and care. Involving patients and carers aims to be empowering and to promote participation in decision-making (Sykes and Goodwin 2007), and patients' involvement in their health care has been associated with better health outcomes (Arnetz et al. 2008). The notion of partnership implies an equal relationship, underpinned by mutual respect, and should lead to greater empowerment of people accessing health care and more effective self-management. Values underpinning partnership working relate closely to those that underlie person-centred approaches (Chapter 7) and to promoting dignity in care (Chapter 6). This chapter focusses on partnership working and related concepts with application to a range of practice examples.

Learning outcomes

By the end of this chapter, you will be able to

- Explore the nature and benefits of partnership working with people who access health care;
- Analyse key aspects of partnership working, including relationships, shared decision-making and empowerment;
- Reflect on personal experiences and practice in relation to partnership working.

The nature and benefits of partnership working

The Nursing and Midwifery Council (NMC) (2010) requires that all newly qualified nurses can

> *work in partnership with other health and social care professionals and agencies, service users, carers and families ensuring that decisions about care are shared.*
>
> *(p. 5)*

Partnership working with other professionals is addressed in Chapter 9; this chapter focusses on partnerships with patients/service users, carers and families.

Partnership working is now a well-established goal in health policy generally and in quality guidelines for different fields of health care. The NHS Constitution promises patients that National Health Service (NHS) staff will 'work in partnership with you, your family, carers and representatives', specifying that patients will be involved in their care planning and be provided with information that they can understand in order to participate in choices and decision-making about health care (Department of Health [DH] 2013). Similarly, the Scottish Government (2010), as part of its quality strategy, expressed the aim for

> *mutually beneficial partnerships between patients, their families and those delivering healthcare services which respect individual needs and values and which demonstrate compassion, continuity, clear communication and shared decision-making.*
>
> *(p. 7)*

The Scottish Government stated the intention to 'Support staff, patients and carers to create partnerships which result in shared decision-making'. Partnership working is also embedded in evidence-based guidelines; for example, the National Institute for Health and Clinical Excellence (NICE) (2011) best practice guidelines for improving the experience of people who use adult NHS mental health services includes the standard that healthcare professionals work in partnership with mental health service users and their families or carers. Winness et al. (2010) identified that when mental health service users participate in care processes as equal partners, they perceive that they are viewed as trustworthy persons with dignity and capacity for decisions.

Jonsdottir et al. (2004) highlighted that ethical nursing practice (as explored in Chapter 4) is central to working in partnership. The underpinning values for partnership working are also important to explore.

Activity

Consider the following questions:

- What values underpin partnership working?
- What does it mean to work in partnership with someone?

You probably recognised that respect for others is an essential value in partnership working, and you also might have identified empathy and honesty as important, along with other values. Working in partnership implies a relationship in which each person participates and contributes towards a common goal. It is therefore important in partnership working to mutually agree on a realistic goal and on the roles of each person involved. A partnership should be based on equality and mutual respect, valuing what each person brings to the relationship. From a concept analysis of partnership in health visiting, Bidmead and Cowley (2005) defined partnership in health visiting as being

> *a respectful, negotiated way of working together that enables choice, participation and equity, within an honest, trusting relationship that is based in empathy, support and reciprocity.*
>
> *(p. 203)*

They emphasised that partnership requires a high level of interpersonal qualities and communication skills. Although this analysis was in relation to health visiting, the definition is just as relevant to other areas of nursing.

Gallant et al. (2002) asserted that partnership should lead to client empowerment, which they explained as an improved ability for the service user to act on their own behalf. They further emphasised the need to identify the roles and responsibilities of the partners and that the process of partnership involves power sharing and negotiation. However, in practice, partnership ways of working can be challenging for healthcare professionals. For example, Morgan and Moffatt (2008) studied community nurses' experiences of caring for patients with leg ulcers who they had identified as 'non-healing' and 'non-concordant' with treatment. The findings revealed the expectations of nurses that patients should obey treatment instructions and be positive and participative. The nurses' and patients' goals were not always shared: nurses viewed ulcer healing as the priority, even though this was unlikely, and the patients prioritised achieving comfort. The findings indicated that the nurses did not view the patients in a holistic way but focussed on their leg ulcer alone. When patients tried to exert some control over their own care, nurses viewed them as 'difficult', 'uncooperative' and 'non-compliant'. Morgan and Moffatt (2008) highlighted that at the centre of a successful nurse-patient relationship is a non-judgemental partnership, but that this seemed challenging to achieve especially when ulcers failed to heal, which the nurses found emotionally difficult to handle. The study illustrated that, in practice, partnership working is not necessarily easy and requires non-judgemental attitudes and highly developed communication skills to meet a shared understanding and agreed goals.

Like Bidmead and Cowley (2005), Jonsdottir et al. (2004) emphasised the relational dimension of partnerships. They suggested that in partnership, the nurse and patient need to communicate in a way that is open, caring, mutually responsive and non-directive. They also considered that the nurse must be present with the patient and openly attentive, showing an unconditional warm regard for the person as another human being. They identified the importance of the nurse reaching an understanding of patients' health experiences and getting to know the person involved in the partnership working. In Morgan and Moffatt's (2008) study, the nurses could have focussed more on understanding how the person was living with the leg ulcer and the impact on the person's life, rather than solely on the ulcer.

Partnership working is particularly relevant for people with long-term conditions. As an example, Ingadottir and Jonsdottir (2010) reported on a partnership framework developed for working with patients with chronic obstructive pulmonary disease (COPD). The framework's core principle is an open, caring, mutually responsive and non-directive dialogue between nurses and patients and their families, with a focus on family involvement, assisting with living with symptoms and facilitating access to health care, health being the overall aim. Ingadottir and Jonsdottir (2010) conducted an evaluation of this partnership approach; the results indicated a potential to improve the health of people with COPD and reduce hospital admissions.

Diabetes is another common long-term condition, and nurses in all fields of nursing will encounter people with diabetes. Standard 3 in the National Service Framework (NSF) for Diabetes (DH 2003) concerns empowerment: encouraging partnership in decision-making and supporting people to manage their diabetes and promote their own health. Diabetes UK (2008) reviewed the progress of the NSF and considered that there still needed to be better partnership between people with diabetes and healthcare professionals when planning and agreeing on care. Now, read the scenario in Box 8.1 and consider the questions.

The scenario does not indicate a partnership approach; from Mike's perspective, the nurse adopted a directive and authoritarian manner.

Box 8.1

Practice scenario: partnership working

Mike is 56 years old and has type 2 diabetes, for which he takes insulin. He works shifts, and eating regularly and monitoring his blood glucose are a continual challenge for him. Mike has no other known health problems and keeps physically active. He has smoked for 35 years. He is divorced and lives alone with one adult son. His daughter lives locally and has young children. Mike attends his practice nurse clinic to monitor his diabetes, but his last visit, over a year ago, was not a good experience for him. He told his daughter that he would not go back to the surgery again as the nurse 'told him off' for not monitoring his blood glucose often enough and that she also 'had a go' at him about his smoking. Mike's daughter is trying to persuade Mike to go back to the surgery for a check-up as she is worried about his health. Her grandmother (Mike's mother) has diabetes and had a lower-leg amputation last year.

Questions

1. Reflect on Mike's perceptions of his last visit to the clinic: What characterised the nurse's approach to him?
2. If Mike attends clinic again, how might the practice nurse apply a partnership approach?

As nurses, we need to build a relationship with patients and develop an understanding of the person's world and how we can support them with their health. Cooper et al. (2003) highlighted that people with diabetes need education that will promote their health whilst respecting individuals' self-perceived needs and voluntary choices. They reported on a project to improve education, but they concluded that whilst patients could be educated towards greater autonomy, not all health professionals were ready to work in partnership with them. The study highlighted the importance of clinical staff gaining better understanding not only of diabetes management but also of the theoretical principles underlying patient empowerment.

Abbott and Gunnell's (2005) study of older people with diabetes found that most self-managed their diabetes in the limited sense of self-medication and observing dietary restrictions, and many monitored their blood glucose levels. However, some ignored dietary advice, and although information about diabetes could be helpful, it was also sometimes frightening or confusing. Even though some were extremely independent, several would have preferred more support from health professionals, not finding self-management empowering but a burden. Abbott and Gunnell (2005) concluded that patients who are not given a choice cannot be said to be empowered.

Relationships in partnership working

A successful partnership approach requires a constructive relationship. One conceptual framework for reviewing relationships, used recently by the Health Foundation (2013b) in its examination of health provider–service user relationships, is Wish's (1976) model. The framework has four dimensions, each a spectrum:

- *Power symmetry/asymmetry*: This is the power dynamic of the relationship, or the equality.
- *Valence*: This refers to cooperation versus competition, with the continuum ranging from cooperative and friendly to competitive and hostile.
- *Intensity*: This is the level of interdependence and refers to the frequency of interactions and depth of relationship and commitment of both parties.
- *Formality:* Formality is the extent to which the relationship is social versus professional in nature.

If you return to Box 8.1, you can discern the inequality in the power dynamic of the relationship between Mike and the practice nurse.

Activity

Reflect on your own experiences of power dynamics between nurses and patients/families:

- Who held control and power?
- Why might that have been?

The balance of power in the relationship between service users and healthcare professionals is an important factor in partnership working. Kurz et al. (2008) argued that people experiencing disability and chronic disease often feel powerless, relinquishing medical control to 'more knowledgeable' professionals. Winness et al. (2010) argued that traditionally people with mental health problems have been marginalized and powerless and put into dependent positions. They argued that the philosophy of partnership is based on equalizing power differences, which can only happen when participants are mutually respectful of their humanity. They further proposed that professionals portraying that they attribute 'normality' to service users will start the move away from the power imbalance in professional-user relationships.

In a study of partnership in care in general hospital wards, Henderson (2003) found that nurses understood that involving patients in care required them to give patients information and to share power in decision-making. However, with a few exceptions, most nurses were unwilling to share their decision-making powers, creating a power imbalance and resulting in little patient input. Factors identified included nurses' beliefs that they knew best and that patients lacked medical knowledge, along with the perceived need for nurses to retain their power and maintain control. Patients in the study explained that some nurses tried to persuade them to cooperate; they found that nurses were not prepared to give them information or to listen to their views. Henderson (2003) concluded that if nurses and patients are to work in partnership, nurses must endeavour to equalize the power imbalance; sharing information readily and being open in their communication with patients would be a helpful start.

A number of other studies in different settings have highlighted power imbalances in nurse-patient interactions. Brämberg et al.'s (2012) study of diabetes consultations for people who were immigrants revealed a power imbalance, with the nurse acting as the 'conductor' of the consultation, introducing the topics discussed and giving information. In a study of urgent care experiences, Bridges and Nugus (2010) found that older patients experienced a diminished sense of their individual significance, and a key factor was the imbalance of power between themselves and the healthcare professionals. Also in children's nursing, Corlett and Twycross (2006) identified issues relating to power and control as recurrent themes in much of the literature. They found that, consciously or unconsciously, nurses managed the level of parental participation allowed by controlling the information they gave, the support they provided and the way in which they communicated with parents. Corlett and Twycross (2006) recommended that nurses need to be aware how they interact with parents and the way in which parental involvement can be controlled and manipulated.

From reviewing Box 8.1 in relation to Wish's (1976) model, you might conclude that Mike perceived the nurse to be hostile and unfriendly. Management of long-term conditions like diabetes occurs over many years, giving the opportunity for a positive relationship to develop. However, the actual contact time between nurses and patients may be infrequent and comprise just short appointments. Skills in building a rapid rapport are essential for nurses and other health care professionals in many care settings.

Partnership working is closely aligned with promoting choice and shared decision-making; these concepts, increasingly prominent in health policy, are explored next.

Shared decision-making

Government policy on patient choice and involvement in decisions was set out in the White Paper, *Equity and Excellence: Liberating the NHS* (DH 2010). This was followed up by *Liberating the NHS: No Decision about Me Without Me—Further Consultation on Proposals to Secure Shared Decision Making*, which proposed a model for giving patients and carers more say in decisions about their care and treatment (DH 2012b). NICE specified shared decision-making within the quality standards for mental health care experience (NICE 2011) and patient experience in adult NHS services (NICE 2012).

Activity

Consider:

- What do you think the term ***shared decision-making*** means?
- What do you think would be necessary to achieve shared decision-making in practice?

Various definitions of shared decision-making have been put forward, for example, the Health Foundation (2013a) defined it as

> *a process in which clinicians and patients work together to choose tests, treatments, management, or support packages, based on clinical evidence and patients' informed preferences.*
>
> *(p. 6)*

With a slightly different perspective, and recognising the expertise of all participants in the partnership, Duncan et al. (2010) defined shared decision-making as involving both parties recognised as bringing expertise to the process and working in partnership to make a decision. If you look at Box 8.1, Mike will bring expertise about himself, his lifestyle and his context for living with diabetes. He will know what presents barriers to his diabetes self-management and what helps him to manage his condition. The nurse should bring knowledge of diabetes and its management and how to support patients in managing their condition. Should Mike wish to address his smoking, the nurse should know about smoking cessation resources. So, both parties bring expertise to the situation and should be able to work in partnership to make shared decisions. However, their current relationship does not seem to form the basis for a successful partnership. Duncan et al. (2010) noted that shared decision-making is advocated on the basis that patients have a right to self-determination and that it will increase treatment adherence. If Mike is more involved in decisions about his self-management, they are more likely to be based on goals that he can achieve within the confines of his lifestyle.

As regards what would be necessary for shared decision-making in practice, Dy and Purnell (2012) proposed the key concepts of provider competence, trustworthiness and cultural competence; communication with patients and families; information quality; patient competence; and roles and involvement. Several of these elements seem weak in the relationship between Mike (Box 8.1) and the nurse; for example, trust seems lacking, and communication is not constructive. Entwistle and Watt (2006) argued that current models of patient involvement in decision-making tend to focus on communication within consultations or on the patient's use of information to consider and select one treatment option from a specified set. They asserted that this is a narrow way of working with patients, and they proposed a broader conceptual framework that acknowledges the involvement of patients through what they think and feel about their roles and contributions to decision-making and their relationships with healthcare professionals.

As in partnership working generally, the relationship between patients and professionals remains important. However, an exploration of decision-making in cancer care highlighted a lack of understanding of the significance of interpersonal relationships and interactions in partnership working and the role of the relationships throughout the course of the illness experience (Hubbard et al. 2010). The study also highlighted the important contribution of carers, particularly in relation to information, acting as facilitators during deliberations about choices and supporting patients in decision-making (Hubbard et al. 2010).

A number of other studies have explored shared decision-making in practice. For example, Upton et al. (2011) investigated nurses' perceptions of shared decision-making in asthma consultations. The nurses defined shared decision-making as providing information and offering choice, but this choice was restricted to a limited number of inhalers. The findings revealed that the nurses held the power in consultations, and they viewed shared decision-making as a tool to improve patient outcomes through increased adherence. The authors concluded that shared decision-making was used as a tool to support the nurses' agenda, rather than as a natural expression of equality between the nurse and patient. They also highlighted that, in contrast to the NHS drive towards patient empowerment, the nurses maintained a paternalistic attitude to patients. Upton et al. (2011) argued that there needs to be attitudinal shifts and improvements in knowledge of shared decision-making for the policies to be implemented in practice. They further suggested that if patients are to become more involved in decision-making, nurses will need to be trained to elicit patients' preferences and concerns, develop a better understanding of what shared decision-making and empowerment mean and become willing and confident to share decision-making more equally with patients.

Activity

Reflect on your practice experience and how people were involved in decisions about their care.

- What do people need in order to make an informed decision about their health care?
- Where do you feel the power was held during the process?
- What barriers might there be to shared decision-making?

In shared decision-making, people accessing health care are provided with evidence-based information about options, outcomes and uncertainties, accompanied by support and documentation of their preferences (Health Foundation 2013b). Thus, a key need is information; important considerations relate to the type of information and its accessibility. Following publication of the government's plans for greater choice and shared decision-making, concerns were raised during consultation that some service users, who already find it hard to navigate the NHS, could be further disadvantaged (DH 2012a). There were concerns related to the attitude and behaviours of NHS staff, who may feel that they know best, and that time constraints may prevent health professionals from fully involving the person in decisions about their care (DH 2012a). Some service user groups in the consultation raised that attitudes towards vulnerable groups mean that it is difficult for them to access services; Chapter 1 discussed how organisational culture affects care and highlighted the legal and professional requirement for anti-discriminatory behaviour. Both the Deafness Support Network and the Royal National Institute for the Blind (RNIB) raised that health information is often not provided in an accessible manner; for example, the RNIB pointed out that little information is available in Braille (DH 2012a). Other comments in the consultation related to the reliance on digital information and that not all service users have Internet access or wish to access health information that way.

Activity

Focus on your current (or last) practice learning experience and reflect on access to health information: What information is provided for service users in this setting and how?

- Is it written, verbal or electronic?
- Is it provided in different languages, in Braille and other formats?
- How easy is the information to read? Does it include medical jargon, for example?
- If children or young people access this setting, is the information appropriate for their age?
- Are there any service users who would find the information difficult to access or understand?

Responses to the government's consultation on shared decision-making pointed out that people with lower literacy could be disadvantaged (DH 2012a). The National Children's Bureau (NCB) and Council for Disabled Children highlighted that children and young people wanted better information, explanations and communication and valued being involved in decisions, while pointing out issues of capacity to consent and legal implications (see Chapter 5). In relation to people with learning disabilities, the charity Turning Point asserted that there is insufficient attention to supporting people with learning disabilities to make decisions and that

> *choice and shared decision making can and should be better enabled for people with a learning disability, often involving their families, friends and carers.*
> *(DH 2012a, p. 13)*

In learning disability health policies, promoting choice and decision-making is now a core theme, but in the past it was assumed that people with learning disabilities lacked the capacity to make decisions; their right to make decisions for themselves, as for anyone else, is now recognised (Royal College of Nursing 2011). The Community Health and Learning Foundation highlighted the strong links between health literacy and health knowledge, which is lowest among people with poor educational outcomes, who may be less able to make informed decisions and choices (DH 2012a). Protheroe et al. (2013) explored the perceptions of participation in health care of people with differing socio-economic status, with themes related to health literacy and relationships with healthcare professionals. They found that patients perceived participation in different ways, related to their prior expectations of a healthcare consultation, cultural expectations and social position. They argued that policies aimed at simply improving 'health literacy' and choice will not be successful if other disparities are not addressed.

McCaffery et al. (2010) argued that although there have been major advances in ways to increase patient involvement in health decisions, with the benefits of greater involvement and shared decision-making now widely accepted, there has been little attention given to the development of tools and strategies to support participation of adults with lower literacy, who are members of a group with poor health knowledge, limited involvement in health decisions and poor health outcomes. McCaffery et al. (2010) proposed a framework to consider the different stages of shared health decision-making and the tasks and skills required to achieve each stage.

The Health Foundation (2013a) reported on a selection of improvement projects whereby clinical teams implemented shared decision-making. The report referred to patients who are 'activated': they know how to manage their condition and prevent their health from declining, believe they have an important role in self-managing care and collaborate with providers. The Health Foundation (2013a) identified three questions that activated patients need to ask:

1. What are my options?
2. What are the possible benefits and risks of those options?
3. How likely are the benefits and risks of each option to occur?

Staff participants in the improvement projects highlighted the importance of actively listening to patients and providing information in the context of people's lives rather than giving 'standardised' information (Health Foundation 2013a). Staff also recognised that paternalistic healthcare approaches posed a barrier to shared decision-making, and some struggled with moving away from such approaches. You might reflect on these comments in relation to Mike's experience as discussed in Box 8.1; it seemed that there was little consideration of Mike's shift work in his last practice nurse appointment, and his perception of being 'told off' implies a paternalistic approach rather than one of partnership. The Health Foundation (2013a) also reported that some staff encountered reluctance about shared decision-making from some patients, who were more comfortable with the traditional approach of healthcare professionals making decisions for them.

Gallant et al. (2002) identified that the most frequently cited benefit of partnership is empowerment of service users; this concept is explored next.

Empowerment

Holmström and Röing (2012) asserted that empowerment offers opportunities for patients to increase their autonomy and involvement in their care and treatment. Grealish et al. (2013) reported that there is evidence that empowerment is central to improving the effectiveness and quality of mental health care, increasing involvement, choice and access to health information for service users. They further asserted that through the process of empowerment, people may better understand their health needs and accordingly improve their prognoses.

Following a concept analysis, Dowling et al. (2011) identified that empowerment is fundamental to the self-management of any chronic illness but that nurses and service users require skills and self-awareness to engage in the empowerment process. They suggested that the first step in the empowerment process in chronic illness is that nurses need to surrender control. Both nurses and patients need to be able to communicate effectively. Nurses themselves need to feel empowered and focus on the client's goals; patients need to be willing to participate in change and to engage actively with the empowerment process (Dowling et al. 2011). Dowling et al. (2011) further argued that central to the empowerment process in chronic illness is having a clinical environment which nurtures trust and reciprocity between the nurse and client, and sufficient time to allow this. From this analysis, it is clear that empowerment is influenced by a complex interrelationship between nurse, patient and care environment.

Although empowerment seems well accepted as an important principle in health care, there are varying experiences in practice. Grealish et al. (2013) studied empowerment from the perspective of young people experiencing psychosis, finding that they conceptualized empowerment as being listened to, being understood, taking control and making decisions for themselves. Young people placed high importance on experiencing personal empowerment as users of mental health services, and they considered being empowered as the most important factor for determining their own recovery. However, the young people viewed mental health workers as varying in their ability and willingness to address and help facilitate empowerment. Grealish et al. (2013) suggested that clinicians must consider whose needs are being met when decisions are made for young people with psychosis.

Asimakopoulou et al. (2012) explored what healthcare professionals working with people with diabetes understood by the term *empowerment*, their attitudes towards it and whether they believed they practised in ways consistent with empowerment principles. They found that there was no clear specific understanding of what empowerment is and what it involves, although there was broad reporting of factors concerning education and informed choices. Healthcare professionals disagreed about the level of freedom patients should have in making choices–from leading them to the 'right' choice to an acceptance that patients may have the right to choose not to be empowered. They believed there was resistance from some patients to the process of empowerment as part of active partnership in care. They concluded that although empowerment is a popular concept in theory, its practical, everyday implementation in practice can be problematic.

The Expert Patients Programme

Education and information are essential for empowerment. The Expert Patients Programme provides free self-management courses for people living with any long-term health condition. The courses provide tools and techniques to help patients manage their conditions better and provide information about making informed choices and working in partnership with healthcare professionals. The programme is well established and has been evaluated, indicating positive effects on patients and economic benefits (Expert Patients Programme 2010).

Activity

Access the Expert Patients Programme website (http://www.expertpatients.co.uk/course-participants/personal-stories) and read some of the personal stories from people who have been involved and the impact on their lives. There are personal accounts from a range of people, some with mental health conditions and others living with physical health conditions such as multiple sclerosis (MS).

Partnerships with families

In Chapter 7, we explored family-centred care. A central attribute of family-centred care is a partnership between parents and professionals, with core values of mutuality and common goals, shared responsibility, parent autonomy and control, negotiation and family support (Mikkelsen and Frederiksen 2011). Kenyon and Barnett (2001) described that a jointly managed plan of care, which actively involved the child and family in identifying the partnership in care component, is essential. However, they suggested that a major culture change is needed to ensure a shift in the balance of power for nursing care delivery away from the children's nurse towards the child/parent/carer.

In Australia and New Zealand, the family partnership model has been widely implemented in child and family health services. In an investigation of what the model's application means in day-to-day practice, Fowler et al. (2012) found it was well received and increased health professionals' confidence in their approach to working with parents.

Whilst much of the literature on partnership working with families focusses on parents of children accessing health care, partnership working is equally relevant to families of adults with long-term conditions, as for many people, family carers play a crucial role. There are over 6 million unpaid carers in the United Kingdom who help family, friends or neighbours with care because of the health issues of these family, friends or neighbours (Buckner and Yeandle 2011), so nurses working with people with long-term health conditions should be developing partnerships with carers along with the patient.

Partnership working and service development

This chapter has so far focussed on partnership working between healthcare professionals and service users and families to empower individuals to manage their health. However, partnership working is also essential for developing services that best meet the needs of people accessing health care and their families. NHS trust and other healthcare providers are increasingly working in partnership with their local communities and with service user groups. The Health and Social Care Act (DH 2012) established health and well-being boards as a forum where key leaders from the health and care system can work together to improve the health and well-being of their local population and reduce health inequalities. The boards were established in April 2013; it is expected that the membership will include service user representatives. Each board will have a local Healthwatch representative member who will have a formal role in involving the public in major decision-making concerning local health and social care; this work is expected to feed into the health and well-being boards. Thus, these structures should facilitate local involvement of the public in health and social care service development.

Activity

Find out how your local NHS trust works in partnership.

- Look on the website: What evidence is there of partnership working with service users and the public?
- Do any of the specialist nurses you have worked with, or unit or ward staff, work with service user groups (e.g. Diabetes UK, Age UK, Mind)?

You may have found out about patient experience or similar groups in NHS trusts. They are likely to have representation on NHS trust boards and participate in trust activity, particularly quality monitoring and service development. Nurses working in specialist services often work in close partnership with service user groups. Box 8.2 provides an example of a successful new service developed in a partnership between a nursing team and people with MS.

National Voices is a coalition of health and social care charities, which aims that individuals, families and communities are involved in all decisions about health and care–from individual treatment decisions to major service design, and including research. National Voices is working to ensure that patient and public involvement are properly embedded in the new commissioning structures in England and in the implementation of the DH's information strategy to ensure that people have the information they need to make informed choices about their health and treatment and access to their health records. National Voices is campaigning for the active involvement of volunteers, voluntary organisations and groups

Box 8.2

Example of partnership working for service development

Multiple sclerosis is a long-term neurological condition that affects 100,000 people in the United Kingdom (http://www.mssociety.org.uk/what-is-ms). The MS nursing team at the National Hospital for Neurology and Neurosurgery, University College London Hospitals (UCLH), provides care in the biggest MS unit in the country. Every year, some 3,000 people with MS use the services. The nursing team recognised that patient access to services was difficult as nurse specialists were hard to reach. Patients were given a telephone number, but most of the time it went straight to an answer phone as the nurses were busy delivering care in clinics. This was frustrating for both the patients and the nurses.

The nursing team audited the service and asked patients about their level of satisfaction. Patients indicated that when they were in clinic the service was excellent; however; as guessed, the problem was trying to obtain advice between clinic appointments. The level of satisfaction with access was low at 49%.

The nursing team wanted to improve this and secured funding to pilot and test a new telephone advice line called NeuroDirect. During the pilot, the line was manned continuously during office hours from Monday to Friday. The aim was that patients could have their queries or problems dealt with immediately without having to wait for a clinician to call them back.

Before the pilot, the nursing team asked people with MS what they would want from the service. Patients indicated their priorities: It was important that the nurses on NeuroDirect

- Were caring and showed concern
- Had listening skills
- Had access to the person's medical history
- Were clear communicators
- Collaborated with patients to make decisions
- Collaborated with other team members
- Were competent in management of MS
- Responded to their concerns
- Treated each person as an individual
- Shared knowledgeable advice
- Informed the person of options and alternatives
- Engaged the individual person in treatment decisions
- Reassured and helped build the person's confidence.

Continued

Box 8.2 (*Continued*)

Example of partnership working for service development

The information from the patients was used to design and deliver the service that people wanted. Patient feedback on the new service was great: people liked being able to speak to a person rather than an answering machine, being able to get through immediately, not having to wait anxiously for a day or more for a response and obtaining immediate feedback about their problem. Comments included the following:

> *[Their] knowledge is good and I like that it's personal and nurses know my details.*
>
> *The service is excellent and people really do need it. The team have always been wonderful but now I can speak directly to them when needed.*

NeuroDirect is now embedded as a service in UCLH and deals with approximately 100 people per week. The best news is that patient satisfaction is now 93%, an example of how simply asking and listening to your patients can improve care.

Bernadette Porter
Consultant Nurse, Multiple Sclerosis, University College London Hospitals

of service users in the design and delivery of services. You can find out more about the work of National Voices from its website (http://www.nationalvoices.org.uk/).

Learning disability partnership boards should be set up locally and work in partnership with people with learning disabilities and their families. The NHS Confederation (2011) published operating principles for these boards, which should have an important role in driving local change and improvements. Their roles include assessing and benchmarking progress and influencing local strategic planning and commissioning. The boards should ensure that people with learning disabilities and their family carers are fully involved in decision-making for local services. As an example from learning disability services, Roberts et al. (2012) reported on partnership working with a group of NHS service users in a project that was designed to increase their knowledge of human rights, as part of a broader set of initiatives focussing on changing organisational culture. During the project, 'co-production' emerged as the preferred model for promoting service users' understandings of human rights and resolving dilemmas about services being empowering. The project led to the sharing of service design and delivery more equally with service users. Roberts et al. (2012) concluded that combining service user involvement with a human rights-based approach could lead to a move away from tokenism towards collaboration, empowerment and redistribution of power.

Chapter summary

This chapter focussed on the expectation that nurses will work in partnership with people who are accessing healthcare needs, families and communities. There is now a central theme of partnership and shared decision-making in healthcare policy: no decision about me without me. This presents a distinct move away from traditional, hierarchical and paternalistic approaches to health care that dominated previously. However, for partnership working in health care to become a reality, healthcare staff, including nurses, need appropriate values, attitudes and skills for working with service users and carers so that they can build trusting relationships based on mutual respect. The shift to partnership working may also take some adjustment for health service users, as people with long-standing experience of health care may have developed expectations of professionals directing their care and making health decisions for them. As well as a move towards partnership working with individual service users, involvement of service users in health service development is an important consideration and should become a central feature across health care.

References

Abbott, S., Gunnell, C. 2005. Are older people with diabetes compliant or empowered? *Practice Nursing* 16(11): 560–564.

Arnetz, J.E., Winblad, U., Arnetz, B.B., Höglund, A.T. 2008. Physicians' and nurses' perceptions of patient involvement in myocardial infarction care. *European Journal of Cardiovascular Nursing* 7(2): 113–120.

Asimakopoulou, K., Newton, P., Sinclair, A.J., Scambler, S. 2012. Health care professionals' understanding and day-to-day practice of patient empowerment in diabetes; Time to pause for thought? *Diabetes Research & Clinical Practice* 95(2): 224–229.

Bidmead, C., Cowley, S. 2005 A concept analysis of partnership with clients. *Community Practitioner* 78(6): 203–208.

Brämberg, E.B., Dahlborg-Lyckhage, E., Määttä, S. 2012. Lack of individualized perspective: A qualitative study of diabetes care for immigrants in Sweden. *Nursing and Health Sciences* 14: 244–249.

Bridges, J., Nugus, P. 2010. Dignity and significance in urgent care: Older people's experiences. *Journal of Research in Nursing* 15(1): 43–53.

Buckner, L., Yeandle, S. 2011. *Valuing Carers 2011: Calculating the Value of Carers' Support*. London: Carers UK. Available from: http://www.carersuk.org (accessed 20 December 2013).

Cooper, H.C., Booth, K., Gill, G. 2003. Patients' perspectives on diabetes health care education. *Health Education Research* 18(2): 191–206.

Corlett, J., Twycross, A. 2006. Negotiation of parental roles within family-centred care: A review of the research. *Journal of Clinical Nursing* 15(10): 1308–1316.

Department of Health. 2003. *National Service Framework for Diabetes: Delivery Strategy*. London: DH.

Department of Health. 2010. *Equity and Excellence: Liberating the NHS*. Available from: https://www.gov.uk/government/uploads/system/uploads/attachment_data/file/213823/dh_117794.pdf (accessed 1 November 2013).

Department of Health. 2012a. *Equality Analysis: Government Response to: Liberating the NHS—No Decision about me, Without Me*. Available from: https://www.gov.uk/government/uploads/system/uploads/attachment_data/file/156259/Equality-Analysis-no-decision-about-me-without-me.pdf.pdf (accessed 2 November 2013).

Department of Health. 2012b. *Liberating the NHS: No Decision about Me Without Me—Further Consultation on Proposals to Secure Shared Decision Making*. Gateway reference 18444. Available from: https://www.gov.uk/government/uploads/system/uploads/attachment_data/file/216980/Liberating-the-NHS-No-decision-about-me-without-me-Government-response.pdf (accessed 1 November 2013).

Department of Health. 2013. *The NHS Constitution for England*. Available from: https://www.gov.uk/government/publications/the-nhs-constitution-for-england (accessed 24 November 2013).

Diabetes UK. 2008. *The National Service Framework (NSF) for Diabetes: Five Years On. Are We Half Way There?* Available from: http://www.diabetes.org.uk/Documents/Reports/Five_years_on_-_are_we_half_way_there2008.pdf (accessed 2 November 2013).

Dowling, M., Murphy, K., Cooney, A., Casey, D. 2011. A concept analysis of empowerment in chronic illness from the perspective of the nurse and the client living with chronic obstructive pulmonary disease. *Journal of Nursing & Healthcare of Chronic Illnesses* 3(4): 476–487.

Duncan, E., Best, C., Hagen, S. 2010. Shared decision making interventions for people with mental health conditions. *Cochrane Database of Systematic Reviews* (1): CD007297.

Dy, S.M., Purnell, T.S. 2012. Key concepts relevant to quality of complex and shared decision-making in health care: A literature review. *Social Science & Medicine* 74(4): 582–587.

Entwistle, V.A., Watt, I.S. 2006. Patient involvement in treatment decision-making: The case for a broader conceptual framework. *Patient Education and Counselling* 63(3): 268–278.

Expert Patients Programme. 2010. *Self Care Reduces Costs and Improves Health—The Evidence*. Available from: http://www.expertpatients.co.uk/publications/self-care-reduces-cost-and-improves-health-evidence (accessed 4 November 2013).

Fowler, C., Rossiter, C., Bigsby, M., Hopwood, N., Lee, A., Dunston, R. 2012. Working in partnership with parents: The experience and challenge of practice innovation in child and family health nursing. *Journal of Clinical Nursing* 21(21/22): 3306–3314.

Gallant, M.H., Beaulieu, M.C., Carnevale, F.A. 2002. Partnership: An analysis of the concept within the nurse–client relationship. *Journal of Advanced Nursing* 40(2): 149–157.

Grealish, A., Tai, S., Hunter, A., Morrison, A.P. 2013. Qualitative exploration of empowerment from the perspective of young people with psychosis. *Clinical Psychology and Psychotherapy* 20(2): 136–148.

Health Foundation. 2013a. *The MAGIC Programme: Evaluation: An Independent Evaluation of the MAGIC (Making Good Decisions in Collaboration) Improvement Programme*. Available from: http://www.health.org.uk/public/cms/75/76/313/4173/MAGIC%20evaluation.pdf?realName=hrsgE6.pdf (accessed 10 November 2013).

Health Foundation. 2013b. *The Puzzle of Changing Relationships: Does Changing Relationships between Healthcare Service Users and Providers Improve the Quality of Care?* Available from: http://www.health.org.uk/public/cms/75/76/313/4177/The%20puzzle%20of%20changing%20relationships.pdf?realName=9RrN28.pdf (accessed 10 November 2013).

Henderson, S. 2003. Power imbalance between nurses and patients: A potential inhibitor of partnership in care. *Journal of Clinical Nursing* 12: 501–508.

Holmström, I., Röing, M. 2010. The relation between patient-centeredness and patient empowerment: a discussion on concepts. *Patient Education and Counselling* 79(2): 167–172.

Hubbard, G., Illingworth, N., Rowa-Dewar, N., Forbat, L., Kearney, N. 2010. Treatment decision-making in cancer care: The role of the carer. *Journal of Clinical Nursing* 19: 2023–2031.

Ingadottir, T.S., Jonsdottir, H. 2010. Partnership-based nursing practice for people with chronic obstructive pulmonary disease and their families: Influences on health-related quality of life and hospital admissions. *Journal of Clinical Nursing* 19: 2795–2805.

Jonsdottir, H., Litchfield, M., Pharris, M.D. 2004. The relational core of nursing practice as partnership. *Journal of Advanced Nursing* 47(3): 241–250.

Kenyon, E., Barnett, N. 2001. Partnership in nursing care (PINC): The Blackburn model. *Journal of Child Health Care* 5(1): 35–38.

Kurz, A.E., Saint-Louis, N., Burke, J.P., Stineman, M.G. 2008. Exploring the personal reality of disability and recovery: A tool for empowering the rehabilitation process. *Qualitative Health Research* 18(1): 90–105.

McCaffery, K.J., Smith, S.K., Wolf, M. 2010. The challenge of shared decision making among patients with lower literacy: A framework for research and development. *Medical Decision Making* 30(1): 35–44.

Mikkelsen, G., Frederiksen, K. 2011. Family-centred care of children in hospital—a concept analysis. *Journal of Advanced Nursing* 67(5): 1152–1162.

Morgan, P.A., Moffatt, C.J. 2008. Non-healing leg ulcers and the nurse–patient relationship. Part 2: The nurse's perspective. *International Wound Journal* 5: 332–339.

National Institute for Health and Clinical Excellence (NICE). 2011. *Service User Experience in Adult Mental Health: Improving the Experience of Care for People Using Adult NHS Mental Health Services*. Clinical guideline 136. Available from: http://www.nice.org.uk/nicemedia/live/13629/57534/57534.pdf (accessed 1 December 2013).

National Institute for Health and Clinical Excellence (NICE). 2012. *Patient Experience in Adult NHS Services: Improving the Experience of Care for People Using Adult NHS Services.* Clinical guideline 138. Available from: http://publications.nice.org.uk/patient-experience-in-adult-nhs-services-improving-the-experience-of-care-for-people-using-adult-cg138 (accessed 1 December 2013).

NHS Confederation. 2011. *Operating Principles for Learning Disability Partnership Boards: Laying the Foundations for Healthier Places.* London: NHS Confederation.

Nursing and Midwifery Council. 2010. *Standards for Pre-registration Nursing Education*. London: NMC.

Protheroe, J., Brooks, H., Chew-Graham, C., Gardner, C., Rogers, A. 2013. 'Permission to participate?' A qualitative study of participation in patients from differing socio-economic backgrounds. *Journal of Health Psychology* 18(8):1046–1055.

Roberts, A., Greenhill, B., Talbot, A., Cuzak, M. 2012. 'Standing up for my human rights': A group's journey beyond consultation towards co-production. *British Journal of Learning Disabilities* 40(4): 292–301.

Royal College of Nursing. 2011. *Meeting the Health Needs of People with Learning Disabilities: RCN Guidance for Nursing Staff.* London: RCN.

Scottish Government. 2010. *The Healthcare Quality Strategy for NHS Scotland.* Available from: http://www.scotland.gov.uk/Resource/Doc/311667/0098354.pdf (accessed 2 December 2013).

Sykes, C., Goodwin, W. 2007. Assessing patient, carer and public involvement in healthcare. *Quality in Primary Care* 15: 45–52.

Upton, J., Fletcher, M., Madoc-Sutton, H., Sheikh, A., Caress, A.-L., Walker, S. 2011. Shared decision making or paternalism in nursing consultations? A qualitative study of primary care asthma nurses: Views on sharing decisions with patients regarding inhaler device selection. *Health Expectations* 14: 374–382.

Winness, M.G., Borg, M., Hessork, S. 2010. Service users' experiences with help and support from crisis resolution teams. A literature review. *Journal of Mental Health* 19(1): 75–87.

Wish, M. 1976. Comparisons among multidimensional structures of interpersonal relations. *Multivariate Behavioral Research* 11(3): 297–324.

9

Working in partnership within interprofessional teams

Introduction

Most people who are admitted into the healthcare system will require the input of one or more health or social care professionals, and this is particularly the case if people have long-term conditions and complex needs. Interprofessional working is therefore essential in ensuring services are delivered in a coordinated way that meets the multiple needs of people accessing health and social care services. This chapter explores the roles and responsibilities of health and social care professionals and agencies involved in delivering health and social care. The concept of collaborative teamworking is explored, as is your contribution to ensuring collaborative working and to making referrals to other professionals appropriately.

Learning outcomes

By the end of this chapter, you will be able to

- Appreciate the range of health and social care professionals and discuss their role in care provision and the concept of shared values and cultures;
- Recognise the need to refer to other professionals to ensure optimum care provision for people accessing health care and their families;
- Reflect on your own care to promote a collaborative approach to care provision.

The development of collaborative working in the National Health Service

Before the National Health Service (NHS) was created in 1948, there were clear divisions between community health, general practitioners (GPs), hospital care and social services, and this continued with the inception of the NHS. This was despite early recognition of the importance of collaborative working in the Beveridge Report of 1942. You can hear Sir William Beveridge speaking on the BBC about his proposals for a new welfare state (http://www.bbc.co.uk/archive/nhs/5139.shtml).

Key reports and documents have been published over the last 50 years that address the need for collaborative working and call for interprofessional teams to provide collaborative care to improve health care and service delivery. For example, the Seebohm Report (1968) recognised that local government services were spread across many departments and suggested that insufficient quantity, inadequate variety and flexibility, poor quality and poor coordination resulted in difficulties for the public to access the help they needed (Seebohm 1968, pp. 29–32). The report also acknowledged three underlying causes for these difficulties: lack of resources, lack of research and knowledge about social needs and the most effective responses, and the fragmented responsibilities between the different departments (Seebohm 1968, pp. 32–35). A proposal was put forward to centralise the various local government welfare services into integrated departments with a central role for social workers. These proposals were established through the 1970 Local Authority Social Services Act.

In 1989, the *Working for Patients* (Department of Health [DH] 1989b) White Paper was published detailing what has been described as 'the most significant cultural shift' (http://www.publications.parliament.uk/pa/cm200910/cmselect/cmhealth/268/26805.htm) in health service reform since the launch of the NHS with the introduction of the 'internal market'. The companion paper to *Working for Patients*, the White Paper *Caring for People: Community Care in the Next Decade and Beyond* (DH 1989a), detailed the way in which community services were to be organised and provided, including a new funding structure; promotion of the independent sector; defining of agency responsibilities; development of needs assessment and care management; promotion of domiciliary, day and respite care; and development of practical support for carers. These White Papers were passed into law by the NHS and Community Care Act (DH 1990). Here, the idea was to put the 'consumer' at the centre of service delivery to pave the way for the ideal of 'collaborative care' between services.

The White Paper *The New NHS, Modern—Dependable* (DH 1997) criticised previous NHS structures, suggesting they had 'stifled innovation and put the needs of institutions ahead of the needs of patients' (p. 14) and that the internal market

> *which intended to make the NHS more efficient ended up fragmenting decision-making and distorting incentives to such an extent that unfairness and bureaucracy became its defining features.*
>
> *(p. 14)*

The White Paper defined a 'third way' of running the NHS which would be based on partnership and would be performance driven, and the collaborative approach to care provision was highly promoted.

So, the development of collaborative working in health and social care continues. The Health Act (DH 1999) dedicated a whole section to partnership between NHS bodies and cooperation between NHS bodies and local authorities. The idea here was to enable services to work more closely together and work more effectively so that provision was more integrated. This has continued to be a theme in revisions to the Health Act. *The NHS Plan: A Plan for Investment, a Plan for Reform* (DH 2000) committed to developing

> *partnerships and co-operation at all levels of care between patients, their carers and families and NHS staff; between the health and social care sector; between different Government departments; between the public sector, voluntary organisations and private providers in the provision of NHS services to ensure a patient-centred service.*
>
> *(p. 5)*

More recently, the Health and Social Care Act (DH 2012) criticised the NHS for not providing integrated services. The act aims to empower patients and put them at the centre of the care they receive by ensuring that care is integrated around the needs of patients. It sets the basis for better collaboration, partnership working and integration across local government and the NHS at all levels. The act seeks to encourage and enable more integration between services and makes recommendations regarding how integration can be strengthened. A number of provisions are set out in the act to enable the NHS local government and other sectors to improve patient outcomes through effective coordinated working.

Therefore, despite the many reforms made to the NHS, as far as collaboration and integrated services are concerned, there are still concerns about standards of care (Francis 2013), some of which could arguably be attributed to a lack of collaborative working.

What is interprofessional working?

A number of definitions of collaborative or interprofessional working exist in the literature. Barrett et al. (2005), for example, took it to mean

> *collaborative practice: that is, the process whereby members of different professionals and/or agencies work together to provide integrated health and/or social care for the benefit of service users.*
>
> *(p. 10)*

Jansen (2008) further defined it as

> *partnerships between two or more health professionals who collaborate to achieve shared decision making according to client-centered goals and values, optimization of the composite team's knowledge, skills, and perspectives, as well as mutual respect and trust among all team members.*
>
> *(p. 218)*

The World Health Organisation (WHO) (2010) defined collaborative practice as that which happens when

> *multiple health workers from different professional backgrounds work together with patients, families, carers and communities to deliver the highest quality of care.*
>
> *(p. 7)*

These health workers could be from regulated and non-regulated professions and may include community health workers, economists, health informaticians, nurses, managers, or social workers.

Over recent years, evidence has increased for the need for interprofessional collaborative working. Day (2013) suggested that there are five drivers for interprofessional working:

1. **The changing health and social care environment**. Patients are being more empowered and more informed and their expectations are greater. Increase in the demand for healthcare services will require different modes of delivery.
2. **Government policy and initiatives**. Government papers have set out to encourage interprofessional working between and within organisations.
3. **High-profile child abuse cases**. Increasing reports of failures in child services indicate a lack of collaboration, poor communication and inadequate training. Chapter 10 gives examples of some of these cases.

4. **Professional developments.** Care provision is increasingly complex, and there is therefore an increased need to expand knowledge and skills of those working in services. Specialist roles are on the increase and often result in the blurring of boundaries between professions, therefore emphasising the need for professional development.
5. **Technological developments**. These have the potential to influence healthcare delivery and mean that healthcare professionals can work more remotely. These developments are needed to ensure that members of interprofessional teams can communicate quickly and effectively across geographical locations.

Interprofessional teams can often be complex because a number of different professionals from a variety of organisations will need to work together. They may have different ideas about the patient or service user and of their needs and the plan for addressing their needs (D'Amour and Oandasan 2005). Grando et al. (2011) echoed this challenge in designing and managing teams of professionals who can collaborate and work together towards a common goal. These challenges can incorporate ambiguous responsibilities and accountability, a lack of continuity due to shift work, a lack of information about an individual's competence that may result in poor organisation of the team, and a lack of clarity about delegation of various tasks or work to individuals (Grando et al. 2011).

With the development of many non-traditional specialist roles in health and social care, there can often be even more blurring of boundaries, and this can cause difficulties when different professional experts present their own philosophical viewpoints about the team. Colyer (2004) suggested that this increase in different professions, with each individual claiming to be equal to the others and claiming to have a unique perspective on care provision, has resulted in an alternative way of making decisions about treatment goals and care processes. In a complex healthcare environment, the interprofessional team needs to work together, be cohesive and open minded to promote a shared ownership so that flexible solutions to often-complex problems can be proposed (D'Amour et al. 2005).

Collaboration is about sharing ideas and taking collective action in working towards a common goal in the interest of the patient (D'Amour et al. 2005). Communication, participation and mutual respect among professionals are essential in the success of the collaborative team (Colyer 2004). Zwarenstein and Reeves (2006) suggested that effective interprofessional collaboration allows professionals to report a patient's condition and need for intervention to another without fear of it being ignored. Under these circumstances, the decision-makers will act and make evidence-based decisions (Zwarenstein and Reeves 2006).

Despite the need to have a shared vision in the best interest of the patient or service user, Freeman et al. (2000) found that having different perceptions of teamwork can hinder professionals when they try to work together. Freeman et al. further suggested that these different philosophies shape the need for a shared vision, the components of effective communication, role understanding and the values of each other's contribution. Freeman et al. (2000, p. 241) offered a description of the philosophies identified in their research:

- **Directive**. Based on the assumption of a hierarchy led by status and power, here the 'team leader' determined 'what, when and how information was communicated and to whom' (Freeman et al. 2000, p. 241). In this structure, those in the lower roles were valued for their service to the higher role. Learning from others was also affected by status, where those in the 'higher' roles felt they had little to learn from those in lower roles and would only learn from their peers or those in even-higher positions. This philosophy was most frequently identified in medical professionals and by some non-specialist nurses.
- **Integrative**. Here, there was a commitment to being a team member and recognition of the different roles and their importance, and an equal value was assigned to each member's contribution. There was also an assumption that team members would learn skills and knowledge from each other. Where this philosophy was shared, it was clear that joint working had developed. This philosophy was most often identified in the therapy and social work professions.
- **Elective**. This was characterised as a system of liaison and related to professionals who worked autonomously, only referring to other professionals when they thought necessary, and communicating with others rather than interacting with others. This was seen to inhibit shared understanding and precluded the negotiation of role boundaries, leading to a distancing from team activities.

Zwarenstein and Reeves (2006) further suggested that if good interprofessional collaboration is evident, and evidence-based decisions are common within the team, the absence of an evidence-based decision by one professional might be detected and intercepted by another. However, this is not possible if the collaboration is poor and relations are hierarchical and marred by conflict (Zwarenstein and Reeves 2006).

Activity

Think about two team meetings you have attended. Which philosophy do you think underpinned these meetings: Were they directive, integrative or elective, and why?

San Martin-Rodriguez et al. (2005) argued that the success of interprofessional collaboration rests on organisational determinants, including human resource management capabilities and strong leadership. They suggested that although numerous structures exist in healthcare systems to promote and encourage interprofessional collaboration to the extent that they are almost mandatory, collaboration in itself is voluntary; that is, participants must be willing to commit to a collaborative process. This willingness can nonetheless depend on the maturity of those in the team, their levels of education and their previous experience of collaborating in this way (San Martin-Rodriguez et al. 2005). They further posited that collaboration is an interpersonal process that also requires trust in each other, mutual respect and communication.

Zwarenstein and Reeves (2006, p. 47) summarised the conditions under which poor interprofessional relationships occur:

- A lack of explicit, appropriate task and role definitions
- The absence of clear leadership
- Insufficient time for team building
- The 'us-and-them' effects of professional socialization
- Frustration created by power and status differentials
- Vertical management structures for each profession

Barrett and Keeping (2005) proposed the following as important in supporting effective interprofessional working:

- Reflection and supervision
- Evaluation
- Education and training
- Reinforcement of professional identity
- Managerial support
- Realistic expectations

In summary, to be successful, interprofessional collaborative working requires professionals to share attitudes, values, knowledge, beliefs and skills based on mutual respect and trust within that team with the common goal of ensuring that decisions are made with the patient or service user at the centre of the care.

Why is interprofessional working needed?

One reason why interprofessional working is needed is that one professional cannot know everything. It is necessary to work with others to deal with complex problems that cannot be resolved by a professional working on his or her own (Hood 2012). However, there are implications that are more serious if there is a lack of coordination and collaboration between professionals. Pollard et al. (2005) suggested that failure to collaborate and breakdowns in communication can have tragic consequences, as revealed in child protection inquiries. Zwarenstein and Reeves (2006) supported this notion by suggesting that failures of interprofessional working have a negative effect on health care and health outcomes and undermine the validity of clinical decisions. Samuelson et al. (2012) argued that the absence of effective collaboration between health and social care professionals could result in patients or carers themselves having to coordinate care. This may not necessarily result in the best outcome for that individual.

The Kennedy report (Kennedy 2001) on the public inquiry into cardiac surgery at Bristol Royal Infirmary highlighted poor organisation, failure of communication, lack of leadership, paternalism and a 'club culture', and a failure to put patients at the centre of care. Following on from such inquiries, interprofessional working is seen as fundamental to improving service quality and safety (Colyer 2004). Gadliardi et al. (2011) further suggested that coordinated, collaborative service delivery reduces mortality, length of stay and readmission to hospital. In addition, they proposed that it improves patient-reported outcomes (e.g. satisfaction and health-related quality of life) for a variety of acute and chronic conditions. People receiving care delivered by a collaborative team reported higher levels of satisfaction with their care, attended fewer clinic appointments (i.e. fewer were necessary because of the coordinated nature of the appointments), presented with fewer symptoms and reported improved health generally (WHO 2010). In community mental health settings, the WHO (2010) posited that the collaborative approach also had a positive impact on the satisfaction of carers, promoted greater acceptance of treatment, reduced treatment duration, decreased care costs, reduced suicide rates, and increased the treatment of psychiatric disorders. Overall, collaborative care improved access to health services and had a positive impact on health outcomes and on patient care and safety.

Ham et al. (2010) provided further evidence that interprofessional working, with good communication and timely transmission of information between hospital and primary care involving health and social care professionals, reduced emergency admissions and use of beds and prevented readmission. In terms of commissioning services, they suggested that accident and emergency (A&E) admissions can be reduced where processes facilitate closer integration with GPs and other services. It would also appear that where older people are assessed as being at risk of admission to the hospital because of avoidable causes, a single assessment and coordinated approach to care reduces hospital stay, A&E visits, risk of falls and delayed transfers (Ham et al. 2010).

As well as having implications for patients and service users, effective interprofessional working has other economic benefits. It is generally acknowledged that there is a diminishing workforce in health care, and this is costly to the health service. It has been suggested that interprofessional collaboration may address this issue by increasing the recruitment and retention of healthcare workers (Bainbridge 2010) and improving job satisfaction (Samuelson et al. 2012).

Your interprofessional learning experience in practice

The results of the Kennedy report on the inquiry into the Bristol Royal Infirmary (Kennedy 2001) indicated that there should be more opportunities for different healthcare professions to share learning, and the Victoria Climbié Report (Laming 2003) identified the need for professionals to understand each other's roles, break down professional barriers and work collaboratively to improve the quality of care. As a result of such concerns, Humphris and Hean (2004) identified the need for radical reform of the education and training of professionals. The reports into the deaths of young children who had been severely abused over a period of time indicated that shared learning is important in the development of collaborative care (Day 2013).

One way of promoting this shared learning is through interprofessional learning (IPL). The literature related to IPL suggests that high-quality care is dependent on practitioners recognising the importance of collaborating within and between teams. IPL is one way of promoting collaboration by allowing professions to work together, learn from others, and support each other with the common aim of enhancing the quality of care provided. Bainbridge (2010) suggested that to reduce errors, healthcare workers must learn how to collaborate with other professionals.

Interprofessional education occurs when 'two or more professions learn with, from and about each other to improve collaboration and the quality of care' (Centre for the Advancement of Interprofessional Education [CAIPE] 2002). Interprofessional education can engender interprofessional capability, enhance practice within each profession, inform joint action to improve services, instigate change, and improve outcomes for individuals, families and communities (CAIPE, 2011).

Many pre-registration nursing courses have IPL strategies embedded into the curriculum, but there is no standardised format. Barr and Low (2012) nonetheless proposed recommendations for integrating IPL into pre-registration education, and CAIPE identified IPL in academic and work-based settings, at pre-registration and post-registration levels, as contributing to the development of interprofessional working skills and the ability to work collaboratively. WHO (2010) suggested that interprofessional education promotes such collaboration because students have the opportunity to review relationships between professions, enhance mutual understanding and explore ways to use their joint expertise in improving the quality of care delivery and patient safety. Barr and Low (2011) also put forward principles of interprofessional education presented in relation to values, process and outcome. Box 9.1 presents the values in interprofessional education.

Activity

Consider the 'values' component of the Barr and Low (2011) principles of interprofessional education presented in Box 9.1 and reflect on how they compare to your own professional values.

Box 9.1

Values in interprofessional education*

Interprofessional education:

- Focusses on the needs of individuals, families and communities to improve their quality of care, health outcomes and well-being
- Applies equal opportunities within and between the professions and all with whom they learn and work
- Respects individuality, difference and diversity within and between the professions and all with whom they learn and work
- Sustains the identity and expertise of each profession
- Promotes parity between professions in the learning environment
- Instils interprofessional values and perspectives throughout uniprofessional and multi-professional learning

* From Centre for the Advancement of Interprofessional Education (CAIPE). 2011. *Principles of Interprofessional Education.* Available from: http://caipe.org.uk/resources/principles-of-interprofessional-education/ (accessed 3 December 2013).

There are many benefits to IPL experiences, including the following:

For you:

- The opportunity to reflect and clarify the role of the patient or service user in your care
- Increased understanding of the value of good teamwork
- Enhanced appreciation of the importance of effective communication across the whole wider team
- Another good opportunity to link theory to practice
- The opportunity for you to interact with other professions
- The opportunity to develop and enhance your teamworking skills
- The opportunity to help you to develop into a competent, qualified practitioner with the skills and knowledge necessary to work collaboratively in a variety of environments

For practitioners:

- The opportunity to share their specialist knowledge and skills with you
- The opportunity to enable them to reflect on their own practice
- The opportunity to learn from you and your experience of interprofessional working
- The opportunity to develop links with other professionals

For service users:

- The potential for improved planning and coordination of their care
- An increased opportunity to understand and contribute to the care they require

You will come across many different roles within health care, but Celletti et al. (2010) suggested that from an international perspective, healthcare professionals do not always collaborate well partly because of the stereotype of their professional disciplines. Whilst you may not be an expert on each of them, IPL should enable you to make links between different professions and services, with the patient or service user at the centre of any decisions made.

You have had the opportunity to think extensively about your own professional philosophy and values in previous chapters of this book. As discussed in Chapter 1, the NHS Constitution sets out common core values that apply to all NHS staff, regardless of their professional background. The Health and Care Professions Council (HCPC), which regulates allied health professions (including occupational therapists, physiotherapists, operating department practitioners) and social workers, provides a *Standards of Conduct, Performance and Ethics* (HCPC 2008), with which all HCPC registered professionals must comply. However, each profession also sets out its own values. To set you on your way to understanding the function and values of different professions, we next consider the roles and values of physiotherapists, occupational therapists, doctors and social workers, as nurses regularly work with staff in these professional roles.

Physiotherapists

Physiotherapists help people of all ages when these individuals are affected by injury, illness or disability, to restore movement and function, prevent disease and manage pain. They facilitate recovery to help people remain independent or stay in work for as long as possible. Physiotherapists work to achieve this in a variety of ways, including movement, exercise, manual therapy, education and advice. At the centre of their work is the notion that they involve people in their own care, through education, awareness, empowerment and participation in their treatment.

The Chartered Society of Physiotherapy (2011) set underpinning ethics, values and concepts for physiotherapy under the following themes:

- **Respect for individual autonomy**: altruism, in terms of giving priority to the interests of individuals
- **Promoting what is best for the individual**: advocacy
- **Avoiding harm**: honesty and integrity
- **Fairness in how services are delivered**: compassion and caring, fulfilment of care and social responsibility, and commitment to excellence
- **Avoiding harm**: accountability for decision-making and actions

Activity

Observe how a physiotherapist demonstrates these values and carries out their role in practice. Note how these values have an impact on a person in your care and on other members of the team.

Occupational therapists

Occupational therapists work in partnership with people who face physical, mental and social disabilities to help them do the things they want to do (including all the activities you would associate with daily living in the home and outside the home) by developing strategies to overcome the barriers to their independence. The strategies may include the use of specialist equipment, and at all times the strategies are based on the person's goals. Occupational therapists work across age ranges; across acute, community and rehabilitation settings; and in a range of fields, including social care, mental health, work rehabilitation, prison care and hospital care. The aim of the occupational therapist is to promote function and quality of life by enabling a person to develop a sense of purpose and identity and facilitating the person in working towards fulfilment of his or her potential.

The College of Occupational Therapists (2010) produced the *Code of Ethics and Professional Conduct*. The areas in this code relate to the following:

- Service user welfare and autonomy
    - Duty of care
    - Welfare
    - Mental capacity and informed consent
    - Confidentiality
- Service provision
    - Equality
    - Resources
    - The occupational therapy process
    - Risk management
    - Record keeping
- Personal/professional integrity
    - Personal integrity
    - Relationships with service users
    - Professional integrity
    - Fitness to practise
    - Substance misuse
- Personal profit or gain

Activity

Observe how an occupational therapist demonstrates these values and carries out his or her role in practice. Note how these values have an impact on a person in your care and on other members of the team.

Doctors

You will meet a range of doctors throughout your career, but they are all governed by the same principles as set by the General Medical Council (2013). In summary, people who require medical care must be able to entrust their lives and health to the doctor who is caring for them. There are four domains to the code of good medical practice:

1. Knowledge, skills and performance
    - Make the care of your patient your first concern.
    - Provide a good standard of practice and care.
    - Keep your professional knowledge and skills up to date.
    - Recognise and work within the limits of your competence.
2. Safety and quality
    - Take prompt action if you think that patient safety, dignity or comfort is being compromised.
    - Protect and promote the health of patients and the public.
3. Communication, partnership and teamwork
    - Treat patients as individuals and respect their dignity.
    - Treat patients politely and considerately.
    - Respect patients' right to confidentiality.
    - Work in partnership with patients.
    - Listen to, and respond to, their concerns and preferences.
    - Give patients the information they want or need in a way they can understand.
    - Respect patients' right to reach decisions with you about their treatment and care.
    - Support patients in caring for themselves to improve and maintain their health.
    - Work with colleagues in the ways that best serve patients' interests.
4. Maintaining trust
    - Be honest and open and act with integrity.
    - Never discriminate unfairly against patients or colleagues.
    - Never abuse your patients' trust in you or the public's trust in the profession.
    - You are personally accountable for your professional practice and must always be prepared to justify your decisions and actions.

Activity

Observe how a doctor demonstrates these values and carries out his or her role in practice. Note how these values have an impact on a person in your care and on other members of the team.

Social workers

Social workers have a variety of roles. They are trained to enhance parenting to support child development, help disadvantaged people, arrange alternative care for children and adults, aid people in poverty, and prevent children from re-offending, to protect the public. The fundamental principles underpinning social work include justice, empowerment, rights and respect. The College of Social Work (2013) developed its own code of ethics for social workers:

- Protect the rights of, promote the interests of, and empower people who use social work services and those who care for and about them.
- Establish and maintain the trust and confidence of people who use social work services and their carers, promoting their independence while protecting them as far as possible from unwanted danger.
- Respect the rights of people who use social work services and their carers, including their right to take reasonable risks, while seeking to ensure that their behaviour does not harm themselves or others.
- Serve, and promote the well-being of, the whole community.
- Promote social justice and display compassion and respect in their professional practice.
- Uphold public trust and confidence in social work.
- Be accountable for the quality of their work and take responsibility for maintaining and improving knowledge and skills.
- Behave in a respectful and collaborative way with other professionals and practitioners who share the duty to promote the well-being of people who use social work services and their carers.
- Support the aims and objectives of the College of Social Work.

Activity

Observe how a social worker demonstrates these values and carries out his or her role in practice. Note how these values have an impact on a person in your care and on other members of the team.

Applying your learning in practice

Having spent some time in practice familiarising yourself with some different professional roles and values, read the two practice scenarios in Boxes 9.2 and 9.3 and carry out the activities. If possible, access students from other professions and carry out these activities together so that you can learn from each other. Also, consider the role of the voluntary sector in your discussions. You could use a template like the one provided in Figure 9.1 to facilitate your discussion about the different roles and contributions within an interprofessional team.

Box 9.2

Practice scenario: interprofessional collaboration in community care

David, aged 35 years, has been prescribed anti-psychotic medication for schizophrenia. He has developed obesity (body mass index 33) and type 2 diabetes because of the development of metabolic syndrome, which was induced by his medication. David is single and long-term unemployed, and he is socially isolated; professionals are currently his sole source of support.

Questions

- Which professionals, and other agencies (e.g. voluntary sector), could contribute to David's care and support? What roles might they play?
- How could these agencies work together collaboratively to ensure that his needs are met and integrate their care effectively?

Box 9.3

Practice scenario: interprofessional collaboration in rehabilitation

Emma is 14 years old and has sustained a spinal cord injury; she is now tetraplegic. Emma's mother tells you that she feels the goals set for Emma by the interprofessional team are unrealistic and that Emma should have more relaxation time.

Reflect on how you could work with the physiotherapist, occupational therapist, sports therapist, teacher and Emma's mother to agree on a suitable programme of rehabilitation with Emma.

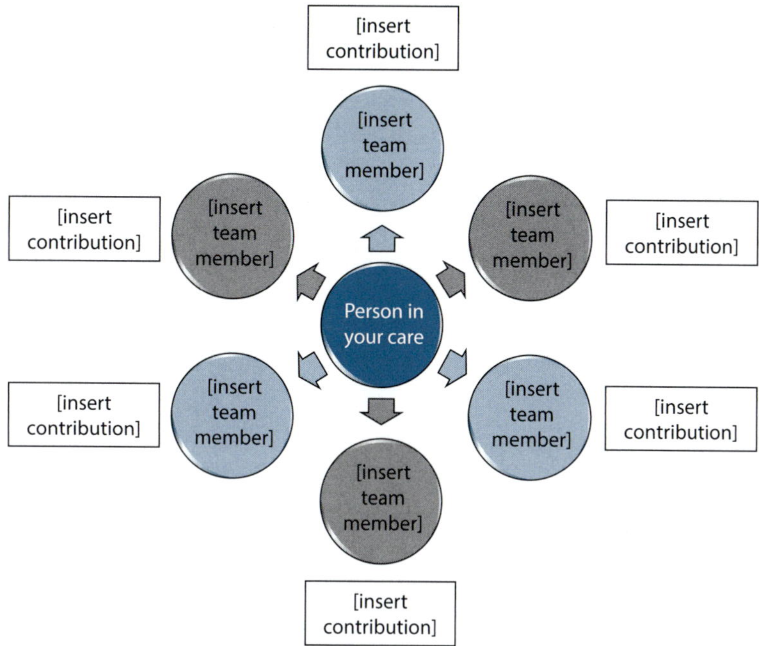

Figure 9.1 Template to record interprofessional collaborative working.

Activity

Now that you have had the chance to learn about individual professional roles, and you have considered a couple of practice scenarios, reflect on your actual experience of working in an interprofessional team and consider whether the following components were evident:

- An understanding of other professionals and their roles and boundaries
- Motivation and commitment to interprofessional working
- Confidence and security in your own role
- Competence
- Good communication and listening skills
- Trust in other team members
- Respect for other professionals
- A supportive and open atmosphere
- Shared power base

- Accountability
- Valuing each other's role
- Organisational support

Finally, judge whether the teams were effective:

- If they were, what made them a success?
- If they were not effective, why was this the case?

Chapter summary

Throughout this chapter, you have been exposed to the concept of working in partnership within an interprofessional team. Definitions of interprofessional working were offered, and the notion of collaboration was explored, as was the need for collaborative working. Throughout your career, you will work with a variety of different health and social care workers, and for interprofessional working to be a success and benefit the person at the centre of care decisions, you need to appreciate and fully understand the roles and values of different professions. You have had the opportunity to start exploring some of these roles and their contribution to interprofessional teams and to the success of the collaborative working process. You should now be more familiar with the concept of interprofessional working and have the knowledge to facilitate your own effective integration into an interprofessional team.

References

Bainbridge, L. 2010. Interprofessional education for interprofessional practice: Will future health care providers embrace collaboration as one answer to improved quality of care? *UBC Faculty of Medicine Medical Journal* 2(1): 9–10.

Barr, H. and Low, H. 2011. Principles of Interprofessional Education: Values. Available from: www.caipe.org.uk/resources/principles-of-interprofessional-education (accessed 19 May 2014).

Barr, H., Low, H. 2012. *Interprofessional Learning in Pre-registration Education Courses: A CAIPE Guide for Commissioners and Regulators of Education.* London: CAIPE.

Barrett, G. and Keeping, C. 2005. The processes required for effective interprofessional working. In Barrett, G., Sellman, D. and Thomas, J. (eds.)

Interprofessional Working in Health and Social Care. Professional Perspectives. New York: Palgrave MacMillan.

Barrett, G., Sellman, D., Thomas, J. 2005. *Interprofessional Working in Health and Social Care. Professional Perspectives.* New York: Palgrave Macmillan.

Celletti, F., Wright, A., Palen, J., Frehywot, S., Markus, A., Greenberg, A. (2010). Can the deployment of community health workers for the delivery of HIV services represent an effective and sustainable response to health workforce shortages? Results of a multicountry study. *AIDS* 24 (Suppl. 1): S45–S57.

Centre for the Advancement of Interprofessional Education (CAIPE). 2002. *Defining IPE.* Available from: http://caipe.org.uk/resources/defining-ipe/ (accessed 3 December 2013).

Centre for the Advancement of Interprofessional Education (CAIPE). 2011. *Principles of Interprofessional Education.* Available from: http://caipe.org.uk/resources/principles-of-interprofessional-education/ (accessed 3 December 2013).

Chartered Society of Physiotherapy. 2011. *Code of Professional Values and Behaviour.* Available from: http://www.csp.org.uk/professional-union/professionalism/csp-expectations-members/code-professional-values-behaviour (accessed 18 October 2013).

College of Occupational Therapists. 2010. *Code of Ethics and Professional Conduct.* Available from: http://www.cot.co.uk/sites/default/files/general/public/code-of-ethics-2010.pdf#search=%22code%22 (accessed 6 December 2013).

College of Social Work. 2013. *Code of Ethics.* Available from: http://www.tcsw.org.uk/uploadedFiles/TheCollege/Members_area/CodeofEthicsAug2013.pdf (accessed 6 December 2013).

Colyer, H.M. 2004. The construction and development of health professions: Where will it end? *Journal of Advanced Nursing* 48(4): 406–412.

D'Amour, D., Ferrada-Videla, M., San Martin Rodriguez, L., Beaulieu, M.D. 2005. The conceptual basis for interprofessional collaboration: Core concepts and theoretical frameworks. *Journal of Interprofessional Care* 1(Suppl.): 116–131.

D'Amour, D., Oandasan, I. 2005. Interprofessionality as the field of interprofessional practice and interprofessional education: An emerging concept. *Journal of Interprofessional Care* Supplement 1: 8–20.

Day, J. 2013. *Interprofessional Working. An Essential Guide for Health and Social Care Professionals.* Hampshire, UK: Cengage Learning.

Department of Health (DH). 1989a. *Caring for People: Community Care in the Next Decade and Beyond.* London: DH.

Department of Health (DH). 1989b. *Working for Patients.* London: DH.

Department of Health (DH). 1990. *NHS and Community Care Act*. London: DH.

Department of Health (DH). 1997. *The New NHS, Modern—Dependable*. London: DH. Available from: http://www.archive.official-documents.co.uk/document/doh/newnhs/contents.htm (accessed 3 December 2013).

Department of Health (DH). 1998. *Partnership in Action: New Opportunities for Joint Working between Health and Social Services*. London: DH.

Department of Health (DH). 1999. *The Health Act*. London: DH. Available from: http://www.legislation.gov.uk/ukpga/1999/8/contents (accessed 3 December 2013).

Department of Health (DH). 2000. *The NHS Plan: A Plan for Investment, a Plan for Reform*. Available from: http://webarchive.nationalarchives.gov.uk/20130107105354/http://www.dh.gov.uk/prod_consum_dh/groups/dh_digitalassets/@dh/@en/@ps/documents/digitalasset/dh_118522.pdf (accessed 3 December 2013).

Department of Health (DH). 2012. *The Health and Social Care Act*. Available from: http://www.legislation.gov.uk/ukpga/2012/7/contents (accessed 3 December 2013).

Francis. 2013. *Report of the Mid Staffordshire NHS Foundation Trust Public Inquiry*. Available from: http://www.midstaffspublicinquiry.com/report (accessed 3 December 2013).

Freeman, M., Miller, C., Ross, N. 2000. The impact of individual philosophies of teamwork on multi-professional practice and the implications for education. *Journal of Interprofessional Care* 14(3): 237–247.

Gadliardi, A.R., Dobrow, M.J., Wright, F.C. 2011. How can we improve cancer care? A review of interprofessional collaboration models and their use in clinical management. *Surgical Oncology*. 20: 146–154.

General Medical Council. 2013. *Good Medical Practice*. Available from: http://www.gmc-uk.org/static/documents/content/GMP_2013.pdf_51447599.pdf (accessed 6 December 2013).

Grando, M.D., Peleg, M., Cuggia, M., Glasspool, D. 2011. Patterns for collaborative work in health care teams. *Artificial Intelligence in Medicine* 53: 139–160.

Ham, C., Imison, C., Jennings, M. 2010. *Avoiding Hospital Admissions. Lessons from Evidence and Experience*. London: King's Fund.

Health and Care Professions Council (HCCPC). 2008. *Standards of Conduct, Performance and Ethics*. Available from: http://www.hpc-uk.org/assets/documents/10003B6EStandardsofconduct,performanceandethics.pdf (accessed 4 November 2013).

Hood, R. 2012. A critical realist model of complexity for interprofessional working. *Journal of Interprofessional Care* 26: 6–12.

Humphris, D., Hean, S. 2004. Educating the future workforce: Building the evidence about interprofessional learning. *Journal of Health Services Research and Policy* 9: 24–27.

Jansen, L. 2008. Collaborative and interdisciplinary health care teams: Ready or not? *Journal of Professional Nursing* 24(4): 218–227.

Kennedy, I. 2001. *Learning from Bristol: The Report of the Public Inquiry into Children's Heart Surgery at the Bristol Royal Infirmary 1984–1995*. London: HMSO. Available from: http://webarchive.nationalarchives.gov.uk/20130107105354/http://www.dh.gov.uk/en/Publicationsandstatistics/Publications/PublicationsPolicyAndGuidance/DH_4002859 (accessed 6 December 2013).

Laming, Lord H. 2003. *The Victoria Climbié Inquiry: A Report on the Inquiry by Lord Laming*. London: HMSO.

Local Authority Social Services Act 1970 http://www.legislation.gov.uk/ukpga/1970/42 (accessed 26 April 2014).

Pollard, K., Sellman, D., Senior, B. 2005. The need for interprofessional working. In Barrett, G., Sellman, D., and Thomas, J. (eds.), *Interprofessional Working in Health and Social Care. Professional Perspectives*. New York: Palgrave Macmillan, 7–17.

Samuelson, M., Tedeschi, P., Aarendonk, D., de la Cuesta, C., Groenewegen, P. 2012. Improving interprofessional collaboration in primary care: Position paper of the European Forum for Primary Care. *Quality in Primary Care* 20: 303–312.

San Martin-Rodriguez, L., Beaulieu, M.D., D'Amour, D., Ferrada-Videla, M. 2005. The determinants of successful collaboration: A review of theoretical and empirical studies. *Journal of Interprofessional Care* 1(Suppl.): 132–147.

Seebohm Report. 1968. *Report of the Committee on Local Authority and Allied Personal Social Services*. Cmnd. 3703. London: HMSO.

World Health Organisation (WHO). 2010. *Framework for Action on Interprofessional Education and Collaborative Practice*. Geneva: WHO. Available from: http://whqlibdoc.who.int/hq/2010/WHO_HRH_HPN_10.3_eng.pdf (accessed 17 October 2013).

Zwarenstein, M., Reeves, S. 2006. Knowledge translation and interprofessional collaboration: Where the rubber of evidence-based care hits the road of teamwork. *The Journal of Continuing Education in the Health Professions* 26(1): 46–54.

10

Vulnerability and safeguarding adults and children

Introduction

This chapter explores vulnerability and introduces you to principles of safeguarding, a concept that is relevant to all nurses in any setting; caring for people who are vulnerable is a fundamental, founding principle of the nursing profession (Dorsen 2010). Training in safeguarding children and adults is mandatory for all healthcare professionals and is an essential element of a nursing course. Health services have a duty to safeguard all service users and provide additional measures for people who are less able to protect themselves from harm or abuse (Department of Health [DH] 2011). Indeed:

> *Living a life that is free from harm and abuse is a fundamental human right of every person and an essential requirement for health and well being.*
>
> *(DH 2011, p. 8)*

Safeguarding applies across settings and disciplines, so interprofessional and collaborative working is crucial (see Chapter 9). This chapter also links closely to other chapters. In particular, Chapter 5, 'Nursing Practice within Legal Frameworks', is highly relevant to safeguarding adults and children:

- The requirements of the Children Act (1989, 2004),
- The Human Rights Act (HRA) (1998),
- The Mental Capacity Act (MCA) (2005),
- The Safeguarding Vulnerable Groups Act (2006).

The chapter also closely relates to Chapter 11, 'Challenging Poor Practice and Raising Concerns', which considers in detail how you can raise concerns about care.

Note: The legislation, government guidelines and policies regarding people who are vulnerable, as well as safeguarding practices, are constantly evolving, so ensure that you continue to update your knowledge in this area.

Learning outcomes

By the end of this chapter, you will be able to

- Explore the nature of vulnerability, with particular reference to people who are accessing health care;
- Analyse the nature of abuse, harm and neglect with reference to children and adults;
- Explain key principles in safeguarding children and adults and the nurse's duty to safeguard those who are vulnerable;
- Reflect on safeguarding of vulnerable people in healthcare practice.

The nature of vulnerability

The term *vulnerability* comes from the Latin *vulnerabilis* and verb *vulnerare*, which means 'to wound' (Dorsen 2010). In everyday life, we use the term *vulnerability* to imply that there is a greater risk of an adverse event; for example, we might refer to a town that is vulnerable to flooding or a shop that is vulnerable to theft. You will also have heard people–individuals and groups–described as vulnerable, both in a general way and concerning specific risks to their health, safety and well-being. De Chesnay and Robinson-Dooley (2012) identified that while many discussions about vulnerability centre on vulnerable populations, as nurses, we must also recognise the vulnerability of individuals. In addition, the individual members of a vulnerable population may not all be vulnerable or view themselves as vulnerable (de Chesnay and Robinson-Dooley 2012).

Dorsen (2010) suggested that the term and concept of vulnerability are used across disciplines to describe the potential for poor outcomes, risk or danger. From a healthcare perspective, vulnerable populations can be defined as social groups who have an increased relative risk or usceptibility to adverse health outcomes (Flaskerud and Winslow 1998). However, as nurses we must be alert to vulnerability from a wider perspective as we may encounter people who are also susceptible to other types of harm. Within society, some people are much more likely than others to be ignored or treated badly because of their vulnerability or because of other people's prejudices (Cowley and Lee 2011).

Activity

Reflect on your practice experiences and people who were referred to as vulnerable and consider:

- Who is vulnerable and why?
- What are people vulnerable to?

In health care, we frequently talk about individuals who are vulnerable in relation to risk, such as their risk of: infection, pressure ulcers, falls, self-harm or deteriorating health status. Many of the risk assessments you will see in practice relate to identifying risk level, for example, the likelihood of a pressure ulcer developing or the risk of a person attempting suicide. The results of these risk assessments should lead to planning and implementation of appropriate actions to reduce risk and safeguard the person.

As well as referring to individuals' vulnerability, we often refer to the vulnerability of certain groups of people, perhaps because they are dependent on other people for essential needs: food, comfort, and protection from harm. Babies and young children are dependent on their parents for almost everything that will keep them healthy and happy. There have been many recent examples reported in the media of sexual abuse of children and young people by groups and individuals in society. Some of these children were vulnerable to sexual abuse not only because of their age but also because of additional factors, for example, they were looked-after children (children in care). In relation to adults in our society, the DH and Home Office (2000) defined *vulnerable adults* as people over 18 years who are unable to protect themselves because of a mental or other disability, age or illness.

Activity

Consider adults you have cared for in practice in the context of the definition of a vulnerable adult. Were any of them vulnerable? Why?

All adults have the potential to become vulnerable at some stage in their lives because of the ageing process or illness (e.g. acute or chronic physical or mental illnesses), resulting in dependency on others for their care needs (Straughair 2011). The Care Quality Commission (CQC) (2013a) recognised that a person's ability to keep themselves safe is partly determined by individual circumstances, and that this may change at different stages in a person's life. Healthcare staff often work with people who, for a range of reasons, may be less able to protect themselves from neglect, harm or abuse (DH 2011). However, some people may be at particular risk as a result of their condition and social circumstances (DH and Home Office 2000; Safeguarding

Vulnerable Groups Act 2006). For example, there have been reports of people with learning disabilities being bullied, abused and exploited by other people in the community (Fyson and Kitson 2010). All nurses must therefore be aware of factors that could contribute to an individual's vulnerability.

The Safeguarding Vulnerable Groups Act (2006), which set out a legislative framework for preventing unsuitable people from working with children or vulnerable adults, recognised the vulnerability of people receiving any form of health care. There are many reasons for vulnerability; for example, some people who have a disability or long-term health condition may need help with moving, eating, and personal care. People with impaired cognitive ability may be less able to protect themselves and are at risk of harm from others. People with dementia, who have physical needs as well as increasingly impaired cognitive ability, may be vulnerable to physical and psychological harm and to other types of abuse and neglect, including financial abuse. People who lack mental capacity are particularly at risk and the Nursing and Midwifery Council's (NMC) (2008) Code requires that nurses ensure that people who lack capacity are fully safeguarded, in line with legislation (see Chapter 2).

Flaskerud and Winslow's (1998) vulnerable populations conceptual model defined vulnerability as the complex interplay between risk, susceptibility, resource availability and health status. They proposed that the level of vulnerability of an individual or group is determined by the interrelationship between these concepts. They highlighted the vulnerability of people who are poor and of low socioeconomic status; those who are at risk of discrimination, marginalisation and stigma; and minority groups. In a concept analysis of vulnerability in adolescents who are homeless, Dorsen (2010) identified multiple factors that increased vulnerability to poor health status and analysed these within Flaskerud and Winslow's (1998) model, modifying it to include people's own health perceptions. They found the model was a useful framework for analysing the vulnerability of groups within the community.

In relation to vulnerable adults, the Centre for Public Scrutiny (2010) highlighted that many disability and user-led organisations view the term *vulnerable* as negative, believing that the term attributes 'victim status' to the person and marginalises the person as a citizen. De Chesnay and Robinson-Dooley (2012) also highlighted that there is a risk that a 'vulnerable population' could become another label and lead to further marginalisation of individuals. An alternative approach is to consider situational circumstances that render a person vulnerable to abuse, rather than the person being vulnerable and therefore being seen as a victim. The Fair Access to Care Services (FACS) framework refers instead to risks to independence and well-being (DH 2010), an approach that is congruent with the government's recent 'personalisation' agenda for the users of public services (Age UK 2012). A consultation on law reform in adult social care found substantial support for the proposal that the term *adult at risk* should replace vulnerable adult and be defined as 'anyone with social care needs who is or may be at risk of significant harm' (Law Commission 2011, p. 146). Nevertheless, the term *vulnerability* continues to be used, so some examples of vulnerability in particular groups are explored next, with a focus on health care. We consider people with learning disabilities, older people, and children, but remember that there is potential for anyone in our society to be in circumstances that increase their vulnerability. In each of the next sections, we explore the complex factors that interrelate to increase vulnerability.

Learning disabilities and vulnerability

Numerous reports have identified that people with learning disabilities are vulnerable to harm, both in the community and in the hospital. The tragic death of Steven Hoskins, a man with a learning disability who was killed by people in his community, further highlights the risk of harm (Cornwall Adult Protection Committee 2007). The Royal College of Nursing (RCN) (2010) asserted that people with learning disabilities belong to one of the most vulnerable groups in society. Jenkins and Davies (2011) also argued that people with learning disabilities have increased vulnerability for many reasons. However, they also highlighted that nurses who work with people with learning disabilities should develop approaches that reduce the need to protect and instead empower people to take control of their own lives.

Jenkins and Davies (2011) identified the numerous factors that increase vulnerability for people with learning disabilities in three groups:

- physical aspects (e.g. frailty, sensory impairment);
- behavioural aspects (e.g. substance misuse, challenging behaviour or aggression);
- social factors, which include social deprivation, poverty, inadequate housing, institutionalisation, communication problems, social isolation, dependence on others for financial/physical/psychological care, and disempowerment in decision-making about their own care.

Discrimination in society is clearly also a factor; Perry (2004) suggested that people with learning disabilities are regularly subjected to hate crimes, for example, being assaulted, shouted at and spat at. The policy document *Valuing People Now* (DH 2009a) emphasised the need to address hate crimes against people with learning disabilities, and the recommendations included improved access to the police and justice system, support, accessible information, complaint procedures and rights of redress.

Although there are undoubtedly many possible factors that increase vulnerability, Northway (2002) argued that vulnerability should not be assumed to be an inevitable part of having a learning disability. Nurses and other healthcare professionals should always approach people as individuals and take a person-centred approach to their assessment and care, without stereotyping or making assumptions (see Chapter 7). However, nurses must be cognisant of factors that increase vulnerability and be vigilant in safeguarding practice. Jenkins and Davies (2011) referred to the 'fine balance between safeguarding people with learning disabilities and empowering them' (p. 38). They acknowledged that frequently people with learning disabilities can demonstrate capability in safeguarding their own interests, but that many do have additional 'vulnerability factors' that warrant safeguarding by professionals, especially when several factors are present. The DH (2009a) acknowledged that avoiding risk altogether would compromise people's choices, and Jenkins and Davies (2011) argued that measured risk-taking is necessary in developing the skills and behaviours that will help a person develop the competence to live independently and raise his or her self-esteem. Furthermore, promoting empowerment and access to advocacy could mitigate against a person's heightened vulnerability (Jenkins and Davies 2011).

The vulnerability of people with learning disabilities is further increased by environmental factors, for example, the culture of organisations that have allowed abuse to flourish (Jenkins and Davies 2011). In 2011, a BBC *Panorama* programme revealed sustained abuse, ill treatment and neglect of people with learning disabilities in Winterbourne View, a private learning disability hospital in England. The subsequent criminal investigation led to six staff being imprisoned (see Chapter 5 for further details). The DH's (2012) report into events at the hospital referred to a 'culture of abuse', noting that: 'Staff whose job was to care for and help people instead routinely mistreated and abused them' (p. 8). The report detailed the failure of different agencies to work together, a factor that has emerged in many previous investigations of abuse of vulnerable people.

People with learning disabilities have also been found to be vulnerable to receiving poor care in acute hospitals. Mencap, a UK charity campaigning for equal rights for children and adults with a learning disability, has reported poor care and treatment of people with learning disabilities, leading to harm and ultimately death in some instances (Mencap 2004, 2007, 2012). Mencap (2012) suggested that such incidents occur because of the lack of value afforded to the life of a person with a learning disability, indicating that discrimination plays a part, despite the Equality Act (2010) and professional codes of practice. The 2012 Mencap report revealed cases in which nurses in acute hospital wards failed to provide even basic care to people with learning disabilities, neglecting nutrition, hydration and pain relief. Clearly in such instances, nurses did not fulfil their duty of care to these patients and safeguard them from harm.

The vulnerability of many people with learning disabilities to physical health problems was highlighted in the Confidential Inquiry into Premature Deaths of People with Learning Disabilities (CIPOLD), which reviewed the deaths of 247 people with learning disabilities in the period 2010–2012 (Heslop et al. 2013). The report revealed the vulnerability of people with learning disabilities because of the multiple factors affecting their health and function. Box 10.1 outlines some key findings from this report. The RCN (2010) highlighted that people with learning disabilities are also at risk of mental health problems; for example, people with autism are vulnerable to developing depression and anxiety disorders.

Box 10.1

Confidential inquiry into premature deaths of people with learning disabilities: some key findings (Heslop et al. 2013)

- In 20 per cent of cases, safeguarding concerns had previously been raised about the person; for a further 8 per cent, safeguarding concerns were raised to the CIPOLD review retrospectively.
- Significantly more (17 per cent) were underweight than the general population (2 per cent), even after excluding those who had lost weight during their final illness.
- Two-thirds of the people who had died lacked independent mobility, half had problems with vision, a quarter had problems with hearing, and over a fifth had problems with both vision and hearing.
- Many had communication difficulties: 30 per cent had limited verbal communication, and 22 per cent could not communicate verbally at all.
- The majority (97 per cent) had one or more long-term or treatable health condition: epilepsy (43 per cent), cardiovascular disease (39 per cent), hypertension (22 per cent), dementia (14 per cent) and osteoporosis (13 per cent).
- More than a third were reported as having difficulty in communicating their pain, but an appropriate pain assessment tool that could have helped had been used with only four people.
- Dependence on others for mobility and eating was significantly more prevalent among those with learning disabilities than a comparison group without learning disabilities.

Older people and vulnerability

In 1991, the United Nations set out principles for governments to adopt for older people in their countries: independence, participation, care, self-fulfilment and dignity. In relation to dignity, the United Nations stated: 'Older persons should be able to live in dignity and security and be free of exploitation and physical or mental abuse' (webpage). However, Tang and Lee (2006) asserted that worldwide, neglect or violation of older people's rights is common, and they argued for the introduction of an international convention on the rights of older people. The Scottish Human Rights Commission (SHRC) identified that older people were an at-risk group in relation to human rights violation in society and launched a project, Care about Rights. The project aimed to empower older people and carers by increasing their awareness and knowledge about human rights, as well as educating care workers (SHRC 2011).

Schröder-Butterfill and Marianti's (2006) analysis of vulnerability in older age identified three components: a complex interaction of specific risks; being exposed to a threat that then occurs; and being unable to deal with the threat because of lack of defence or resource. Brocklehurst and Laurenson (2008) argued that people do not become vulnerable solely because of their older age and that people can become vulnerable at any age. Their analysis of vulnerability in relation to older people raised the concern that the term *vulnerable* can become a label and lead to stereotyping. They argued that while being old in society used to be seen as a sign of wisdom, it is now more likely to be equated with vulnerability and dependence and that discriminatory attitudes to older people contribute to vulnerability. There is, however, substantial evidence that some older people are at risk of abuse sometimes referred to as 'elder abuse'. The charity Action on Elder Abuse (AEA) stated its aim as being to 'protect, and prevent the abuse of vulnerable older adults', and they asserted that by doing so they will 'also protect other adults at risk of abuse' (see http://www.elderabuse.org.uk/). AEA (2012) highlighted that both older men and older women can be at risk of being abused and that abuse can potentially happen wherever they live or visit, including their own home or a carer's home or in a day centre, a care home or in hospital. The prevalence of elder abuse in the United Kingdom is difficult to establish as much may go unreported. However, a survey estimated that 227,000 older people have experienced neglect or abuse by people they should have been able to trust (O' Keeffe et al. 2007).

Many long-term conditions that are associated with ageing affect independence, increasing vulnerability. Examples include dementia, sensory loss, heart failure and respiratory disease, and older people often have co-morbidities. Brocklehurst and Laurenson (2008) identified that as well as physical attributes of vulnerability in older age, there are social (e.g. exclusion, marginalisation), psychological, sexual and spiritual attributes, and further influences are gender, ethnicity and policy aspects. Brocklehurst and Laurenson's (2008) analysis reminds us to view people as individuals and that we should take a person-centred and holistic approach to care for everyone (see Chapter 7).

Many reports have revealed that some older people have experienced poor standards of care in hospitals, care homes and at home (House of Lords/House of Commons 2007; Health Service Ombudsman 2011; British Geriatrics Society 2011). The reports often pertain to poor physical care in relation to nutrition and hydration, personal care, and prevention of pressure ulcers. Recent CQC inspections, focussed on nutrition and dignity in care homes and hospitals, revealed variation in quality of care. While some care homes performed well, in other care homes inspectors witnessed people not being given help to eat and drink or given personal care in a way that respected their privacy (CQC 2013b). In some hospitals, call bells were left unanswered, leaving people without help to get to the toilet and without support for other needs, and patients were not given help to eat and drink (CQC 2013c). There are also examples of abuse from nurses and support workers in institutional settings. Box 10.2 provides an example of the abuse of older people by healthcare assistants in an acute hospital ward; the abuse was only uncovered because student nurses raised their concerns. You might reflect on the accountability of the registered nurses at all levels in this setting and their responsibilities to protect the people in their care under the NMC Code (see Chapter 2). Chapter 11 addresses how to challenge poor practice and raise concerns.

Box 10.2

Example of abuse on an acute hospital ward*

In 2013, three healthcare assistants employed on an older people's hospital ward were found guilty of ill treatment or neglect of a person without capacity under Section 44 of the MCA (2005); one of them was also found guilty of common assault. Two were given jail sentences, and the third was given a suspended sentence and an order to carry out unpaid community work. The women physically and verbally abused the patients, often telling them to shut up, and handled them roughly and aggressively. Other examples of the abuse included holding a sheet over one woman's head and telling her she was dead, slapping and pushing patients. The offences were revealed after a student nurse reported the abuse to senior hospital staff.

* From Mercer, D. 2013. Hospital workers jailed for abusing female patients on Whipps Cross geriatric ward. *The Independent*. Available from: http://www.independent.co.uk/life-style/health-and-families/health-news/hospital-workers-jailed-for-abusing-female-patients-on-whipps-cross-geriatric-ward-8782397.html (accessed 5 October 2013).

Although the example in Box 10.2 clearly constitutes abuse, and we can hope that such extreme examples are rare, vulnerability to indignity in care is more common. Tadd et al. (2011) studied the dignity of older people in hospital using observation and interviews. The research report detailed many examples of lack of dignity for older people; for example, patients who asked to go to the toilet were told to pass urine in a pad instead. The study's findings highlighted the vulnerability of many hospital patients who are dependent on staff to address their fundamental care needs. You might also reflect on the fine line between indignity and abuse, for example, whether being expected to pass urine in a pad constitutes emotional abuse, because of the humiliation of such a situation, as well as indignity.

Box 10.3 provides an example of an older person admitted to hospital from a care home; read this and make your responses.

Box 10.3

An older person's care experiences

Mrs O'Connor, aged 93 years, has Parkinson's disease and was admitted to a trauma ward from a care home after a fall. She was diagnosed with a fractured neck of femur. The nurse from the emergency department reported to ward staff that, on arrival from the care home, Mrs O'Connor was found to have a category 3 pressure ulcer on her sacrum. Mrs O'Connor appeared frail, and her nutritional assessment on the ward confirmed her high risk of malnutrition. Shortly after Mrs O'Connor's arrival on the ward, her daughter arrived. She was distressed and expressed that she was unhappy with the care home. She had looked after her mother herself until 6 months ago, but then her own health problems prevented her from being able to continue. She explained that the care home staff often did not give her mother her medication to treat her Parkinson's disease at the right time, and sometimes they omitted it, saying that Mrs O'Connor refused it. Following surgery to her hip, Mrs O'Connor developed acute delirium. Her daughter visited each day, and on Mrs O'Connor's fourth day in hospital, her daughter found that she was lying in a wet bed and one of her anti-Parkinson's disease tablets was in the bed. She told the nurse that she was not happy with the care on the ward and that her mother was being neglected. She also believed that her mother was in pain.

Questions

- What made Mrs O'Connor vulnerable, and what was she vulnerable to?
- What responses should the ward staff have made in relation to Mrs O'Connor's daughter's concerns about (1) the care home and (2) the care on the ward?

Mrs O'Connor (Box 10.3) was vulnerable because of her Parkinson's disease, a long-term condition that affects the abilities to communicate and to carry out essential self-care and predisposes to falls. Younger adults can also have Parkinson's disease, although this is uncommon. In the care home, Mrs O'Connor's physical frailty rendered her vulnerable as she was dependent on the staff to meet her essential needs for nutrition and hydration, movement, skin care and medication. She was vulnerable to malnutrition, dehydration, pressure ulcers and falls. In the hospital, Mrs O'Connor's vulnerability increased, first because of her injury and subsequent surgery and then because of her delirium, which can develop after surgery or with acute infections, particularly in older, frail individuals and even more so if a person has dementia. Mrs O'Connor's vulnerability was mitigated in part by the advocacy of her daughter, but some older people have no close family members or friends to support and advocate for them, further increasing their vulnerability.

The safeguarding issues that this scenario raises are analysed in more detail further in this chapter. However, the ward staff should be concerned that Mrs O'Connor developed a category 3 pressure ulcer while in the care home and is malnourished; they should raise a safeguarding alert. The care issues that Mrs O'Connor's daughter has raised about the ward care must be investigated. Complaints about care are an important source of feedback, and although the individual's issue must be resolved speedily and trust rebuilt, complaints also offer opportunities for wider organisational learning. For example, the finding of a tablet in the bed is a serious issue; the ward would need to urgently consider how staff help patients to take medication and ensure that all staff appreciate why it is important that anti-Parkinson's medication be given on time. The omission of a prescribed drug is an incident that should be reported. The NHS trust should, however, also consider whether these care issues are isolated to this ward or could apply more widely and need addressing at the institutional level.

Activity

Consider the following questions:

- What response would you make to a patient or family member who makes a complaint about care? Talk to your mentor about this.
- What is the complaints policy in your trust or other organisation? If you are unsure, seek this out on the intranet and familiarise yourself with it.
- How do patients or families know how to complain? Where is information displayed? Look on the trust's website: Could you easily find out how to complain as a relative or patient?

Children and vulnerability

The National Institute for Health and Clinical Excellence (NICE) (2012) guidance for health and social well-being in the early years (under 5 years) includes recommendations for identifying vulnerable children and assessing their needs. The guidance emphasises building trusting relationships with vulnerable families and adopting a non-judgemental approach, while focussing on the child's needs. The guidance outlines a number of factors that may contribute to increasing a child's vulnerability to poor social and emotional well-being.

The deaths of children from abuse by families have led to enquiries, serious case reviews and the development of revised guidelines and legislation on safeguarding (reviewed further in the chapter). You may remember the highly publicised cases of Victoria Climbié (died at 8 years old in 2000), Peter Connolly (died aged 17 months in 2006) and Daniel Pelka (died aged 4 years in 2012). While such cases are fortunately rare, they remind us of the vulnerability of children at the hands of adults who are responsible for their care and protection. The RCN (2007) reported that child deaths from abuse and neglect are not decreasing; there are one or two infants or children killed each week, usually by parents or carers, and infants are particularly vulnerable. Other examples of the vulnerability of children and young people to abuse regularly appear in the media and include bullying and sexual abuse by other children or young people, as well as by adults. Increasingly, the Internet is the medium through which abuse occurs.

The RCN (2007) highlighted that children who cannot easily communicate their distress are at more risk of abuse, and these include younger children, particularly infants, and children who have language problems and learning difficulties. NICE (2009) identified other risk factors as parental or carer drug or alcohol misuse, parental or carer mental health problems, intra-familial violence or history of violent offending, previous child maltreatment in members of the family, known maltreatment of animals by the parent or carer, vulnerable and unsupported parents or carers and pre-existing disability in the child. The RCN (2007) asserted that nurses are well placed to identify children and young people who may be at risk and act to safeguard their welfare.

In many of the highly publicised examples of child deaths, the children and their families had repeated contact with health and social care professionals, and a key factor that regularly emerges is a lack of effective interprofessional and interagency communication, so the full picture of the child's situation is not apparent. The responsibility to recognise children at risk of harm applies to all healthcare professionals, whether their prime role is directly with children or not. For example, nurses working with adults in hospitals or the community should be alert to the welfare of the whole family; they might feel concerned about the child of an adult inpatient or the children of an adult they are visiting in the community. Adults admitted to hospital should be asked about dependents, and nurses should give consideration to potential adverse effects on children if their parent is in hospital. For example, are they being safely cared for by another responsible adult? Likewise, a nurse caring for children in hospital or the community could identify an adult at risk of abuse and should raise concerns.

Definitions of abuse and recognition

This section first considers abuse of adults and then abuse of children.

Abuse of adults

The DH and Home Office (2000) defined abuse as 'a violation of an individual's human and civil rights by any other person or persons' (p. 9). The background to human rights legislation is that in 1948 the United Nations published the Universal Declaration of Human Rights (UDHR), which recognised the 'inherent dignity' of human beings and included the following statement: 'All human beings are born free and equal in dignity and rights' (Article 1). Although the UDHR is not legally binding, many countries have incorporated the UDHR provisions into their laws and constitutions. The European Convention on Human Rights was signed in 1950 and was incorporated into UK law when the HRA (1998) was passed, which recognises that all individuals have minimal and fundamental human rights; see Chapter 5 for further exploration of the HRA and its application to healthcare practice. The DH and Home Office (2000) elaborated that abuse may consist of a single act or repeated acts, it may be intentional or unintentional, and it can cause harm temporarily or over a period of time. The abuse can occur within any relationship and may result in significant harm to, or exploitation of, the person subjected to the abuse (DH and Home Office 2000).

Specifically in relation to older people, in 1993, the AEA established a definition for elder abuse, which has been adopted by the World Health Organisation and other countries across the world and is promoted by the International Network for the Prevention of Elder Abuse. The definition is that it is

> *a single or repeated act or lack of appropriate action, occurring within any relationship where there is an expectation of trust, which causes harm or distress to an older person.*
>
> *(AEA 2012)*

AEA (2012) argued that central to this definition is the 'expectation of trust' between the older person and the other person, but this expectation is subsequently violated. The person abusing the older person could be a family member, friend or neighbour or could be a healthcare worker (as in Box 10.2).

The DH and Home Office (2000) identified six core categories of abuse in relation to adults: physical, sexual, psychological, neglect or acts of omission, discriminatory, and financial or material (see Table 10.1). They also highlighted 'institutional abuse' in relation to repeated episodes of substandard care and poor professional practice within care organisations. Since then, the category of institutional abuse has been increasingly acknowledged. Risk factors for care settings where institutional abuse can occur include a closed, inward-looking culture and weak management at ward and locality levels; a poor institutionalised environment; low staffing levels with high use of bank (temporary) staff; minimal staff development; and poor supervision (DH 2011). In such environments, patients can become de-humanised, and neglect and abuse can remain unrecognised or unchallenged (DH 2011). Age UK (2012) identified that institutional abuse may occur as a result of structures, policies, processes and practices within an organisation, and it detailed examples of such abuse as including toileting by the clock rather than allowing a person to go to the toilet when the person wanted, lack of privacy when attending to people's personal needs, locking people in their rooms, and preventing access to personal belongings.

Phair and Heath (2012) identified that the broadening scope of the safeguarding agenda now includes domestic abuse, forced marriage

Table 10.1 Types of Abuse and Examples

Type of abuse	Examples
Physical	Hitting, slapping, pushing, kicking, misuse of medication, restraint, or inappropriate sanctions
Sexual	Rape and sexual assault or sexual acts to which the vulnerable adult has not consented, could not consent or was pressured into consenting
Psychological	Emotional abuse, threats of harm or abandonment, deprivation of contact, humiliation, blaming, controlling, intimidation, coercion, harassment, verbal abuse, isolation or withdrawal from services or supportive networks
Financial and material	Theft; fraud; exploitation; pressure in connection with wills, property or inheritance or financial transactions; or the misuse or misappropriation of property, possessions or benefits
Neglect and acts of omission	Ignoring medical or physical care needs; failure to provide access to appropriate health, social care or educational services; the withholding of the necessities of life, such as medication, adequate nutrition and heating
Discriminatory	Racist; sexist; that based on a person's disability; and other forms of harassment, slurs or similar treatment

Source: Department of Health (DH) and Home Office. 2000. *No Secrets: Guidance on Developing and Implementing Multi-Agency Policies and Procedures to Protect Vulnerable Adults From Abuse.* London: DH, p. 9.

and hate crime. They argued that failure to work in a person's best interest and follow the principles outlined in the MCA (2005) may also be deemed to be abuse, and prosecution may result.

Activity

Look at Table 10.1: What types of abuse did the patients mentioned in Boxes 10.2 and 10.3 experience?

Now, look again at Table 10.1. For each type of abuse, consider the following: How would you recognise that a person was experiencing abuse?

Looking at Box 10.2, the healthcare assistants' abuse of the patients on this hospital ward was both physical and emotional. Mrs O'Connor's category 3 pressure ulcer and her malnutrition (Box 10.3) could be caused by neglect or acts of omission; an investigation of the care delivered would clarify this. A key aspect would be the care home's records of her pressure area, risk assessment and prevention measures, and nutrition provided. There is insufficient information regarding whether she experienced other types of abuse at the care home. In the hospital ward, Mrs O'Connor's daughter's complaint needs investigating; failure to promptly deal with a patient's incontinence and lack of administration of medication could both be considered neglect or acts of omission as well.

To safeguard vulnerable adults, nurses need to understand the different types of adult abuse and the associated signs and symptoms, ensuring that any abuse is reported appropriately (Straughair 2011). Some types of abuse can be easier to recognise than others; Table 10.2 sets out examples of when you might suspect abuse, but the key point is to be

Table 10.2 Recognition of Abuse

Type of abuse	Recognition
Physical	Bruising (which may be new or old), burns, unexplained minor injuries, fractures, malnourishment and marks associated with physical restraint
Sexual	Over-sexualised behaviour, pain, itching, bruising or bleeding in the genital area, recurrent urinary tract infection and sexually transmitted infection
Psychological	Depression, withdrawal, low self-esteem, attention-seeking behaviour and changes in behaviour or personality
Neglect and acts of omission	Poor physical condition or appearance, unexplained weight loss, malnutrition, dehydration, pressure ulcers
Financial	Inability to pay bills or purchase adequate food; neglected, unkempt or malnourished appearance; and unusual bank account activity

alert and vigilant. Abuse that is not witnessed can be difficult to detect. It is important to listen to the person concerned, but many people who are particularly susceptible to abuse are those who will have difficulty communicating, for example, the patients mentioned in Box 10.2 were frail and had dementia. In the example given previously of the abuse of people with learning disabilities at Winterbourne View, the residents had learning disabilities, and despite many of them attending the local accident and emergency department with injuries and the police being called in to the hospital regularly to deal with incidents, the abuse was only brought to light through an undercover investigation by BBC's *Panorama* after a staff member from Winterbourne View contacted them.

Abuse of children

The document *Working Together to Safeguard Children: A Guide to Inter-agency Working to Safeguard and Promote the Welfare of Children* (HM Government 2013) set out definitions for abuse, and the different types of abuse, in relation to children (see Table 10.3). Read the table carefully and in particular pay attention to the detailed definition of emotional abuse, which recognises that the other types of abuse will inevitably also include emotional abuse. In the examples of child death referred to previously (e.g. of Daniel Pelka), the children concerned had usually suffered neglect (e.g. withholding of food) as well as physical and emotional abuse.

Recognition of signs and symptoms of abuse is an essential first stage in safeguarding children (Thornberry 2010), but as with adults, it is not always clear-cut, especially as perpetrators of abuse often go to considerable lengths to prevent the abuse from coming to light or provide explanations in a plausible way. For example, when Daniel Pelka's schoolteachers raised concerns with his mother that Daniel was always hungry and was taking food out of bins at school, his mother replied that he had a health problem (Coventry Safeguarding Children Board 2013). The NICE (2009) guidelines referred to the 'alerting features' that healthcare professionals should be aware of in relation to child maltreatment. They recommended that health professionals take a systematic approach and

1. Listen and observe, drawing on the full range of information from different sources;
2. Seek an explanation for any injury or presentation from both the parent or carer and the child or young person in an open and non-judgemental manner;
3. Record what they have observed or heard and why this is of concern;
4. Consider, suspect or exclude maltreatment and report to a more senior colleague.

Table 10.3 Definitions of Abuse and Neglect in Children

Type of abuse	Explanation
Abuse	A form of maltreatment of a child. Somebody may abuse or neglect a child by inflicting harm or by failing to act to prevent harm. Children may be abused in a family or in an institutional or community setting by those known to them or, more rarely, by others (e.g. via the Internet). They may be abused by an adult or adults or by another child or children.
Physical abuse	A form of abuse that may involve hitting, shaking, throwing, poisoning, burning or scalding, drowning, suffocating or otherwise causing physical harm to a child. Physical harm may also be caused when a parent or carer fabricates the symptoms of, or deliberately induces, illness in a child.
Emotional abuse	The persistent emotional maltreatment of a child such as to cause severe and persistent adverse effects on the child's emotional development. It may involve conveying to a child that the child is worthless or unloved, inadequate, or valued only insofar as the child meets the needs of another person. It may include not giving the child opportunities to express his or her views, deliberately silencing the child or 'making fun' of what the child says or how the child communicates. It may feature age or developmentally inappropriate expectations being imposed on children. These may include interactions that are beyond a child's developmental capability, as well as overprotection and limitation of exploration and learning, or preventing the child participating in normal social interaction. It may involve seeing or hearing the ill treatment of another. It may involve serious bullying (including cyberbullying), causing children frequently to feel frightened or in danger, or the exploitation or corruption of children. Some level of emotional abuse is involved in all types of maltreatment of a child, although it may occur alone.
Sexual abuse	Involves forcing or enticing a child or young person to take part in sexual activities, not necessarily involving a high level of violence, whether or not the child is aware of what is happening. The activities may involve physical contact, including assault by penetration (e.g. rape or oral sex) or non-penetrative acts such as masturbation, kissing, rubbing and touching outside of clothing. They may also include non-contact activities, such as involving children in looking at, or in the production of, sexual images, watching sexual activities, encouraging children to behave in sexually inappropriate ways, or grooming a child in preparation for abuse (including via the Internet). Sexual abuse is not solely perpetrated by adult males. Women can also commit acts of sexual abuse, as can other children.

Continued

Table 10.3 (*Continued*) Definitions of Abuse and Neglect in Children

Type of abuse	Explanation
Neglect of their responsibilities	The persistent failure to meet a child's basic physical or psychological needs, likely to result in the serious impairment of the child's health or development. Neglect may occur during pregnancy as a result of maternal substance abuse. Once a child is born, neglect may involve a parent or carer failing to • provide adequate food, clothing and shelter (including exclusion from home or abandonment); • protect a child from physical and emotional harm or danger; • ensure adequate supervision (including the use of inadequate caregivers); or • ensure access to appropriate medical care or treatment. It may also include neglect of, or unresponsiveness to, a child's basic emotional needs.

Source: HM Government. 2013. *Working Together to Safeguard Children: A Guide to Inter-agency Working to Safeguard and Promote the Welfare of Children.* pp. 85–86. Available from: http://www.education.gov.uk/aboutdfe/statutory/g00213160/working-together-to-safeguard-children (accessed 14 October 2013).

Activity

Look at Table 10.3 and consider how you might recognise these forms of abuse in children.

Now, access the NICE (2009) guidelines on recognition of maltreatment* of children (http://publications.nice.org.uk/when-to-suspect-child-maltreatment-cg89/guidance). Use these guidelines to make brief notes on how you might recognise abuse.

* Abuse is a form of maltreatment (DH 2013).

If you have any concerns about the welfare of a child or adult, you must raise these with a staff member. Vigilance and recognition of possible abuse are crucial in safeguarding practices.

Safeguarding

The CQC (2013a) uses the term *safeguarding* in relation to

> *a range of activities that organisations should have in place to protect people (both children and adults) whose circumstances make them particularly vulnerable to abuse, neglect or harm.*
>
> *(p. 3)*

The CQC (2013a) further emphasises that safeguarding is the responsibility of whole communities and that it

> *depends on the everyday vigilance of everyone who plays a part in the lives of children or adults in vulnerable situations to ensure that people are kept as safe from harm as possible.*
>
> *(p. 4)*

Read the scenario in Box 10.4 and reflect on the questions posed. In relation to question 1, you may wish to refer to the previous section that explored vulnerability, and the NICE (2009) guidelines may be helpful for recognising maltreatment of children.

Box 10.4

Practice scenario: safeguarding a family in practice

Nadia is 36 years old and was admitted to an acute mental health unit under the Mental Health Act (Section 2). She has a long history of depression, since the birth of her first child, and is currently severely depressed and suicidal. During her initial assessment, she revealed that she has been physically abused by her partner, but she does not wish to report this to the police. She has an 8-year-old daughter and a 10-year-old son, who are at home with her partner. When he brings the children in to visit later that day, they are quiet and withdrawn. The little girl's hair looks matted, and the children look dishevelled. You feel concerned about the welfare of Nadia and her children.

Questions

1. What safeguarding issues might there be in relation to Nadia and her family?
2. What would you do about your concerns?
3. What support would you offer Nadia?

The scenario in Box 10.4 raises safeguarding concerns about both Nadia and her children. You would need to follow your organisation's safeguarding policies.

Activity

What do you know about the safeguarding structures and policies in your organisation?

Identify the following:

1. Who are the named leads for safeguarding adults and children?
2. Access your organisation's policies for adult and child safeguarding and related documents. Look for adult safeguarding alert forms and flowcharts to aid decision-making.
3. Consider how the policies and documents might help you deal with safeguarding issues, as raised in Box 10.4.

Your actions are likely to include reporting your concerns to your manager and the social work team; instigating child protection procedures for Nadia's children, according to trust policy; and submitting a completed safeguarding adults alert form. After initial assessment and confirmation that there is a safeguarding issue, the alert will be referred to an adult protection coordinator who is a member of the adult safeguarding board. You must record factually and accurately what Nadia said to you in her notes, any injuries she showed you and what you observed about the children. You should inform the doctor who will examine Nadia for any injuries, which must be fully documented. You will need to be reassuring, honest and supportive to Nadia about the need to take safeguarding action. It would be important to find out if there are other family members who could support the family. Dealing with such situations can be distressing for staff; ensure you talk to your mentor or personal tutor if you need support.

The next sections explore the following in more detail: safeguarding adults, which will include a subsection on the Deprivation of Liberty Safeguards (DOLS), and safeguarding children. The sections refer to relevant legislation and guidance, most of which is specific to children or adults. However, the Safeguarding Vulnerable Groups Act (2006) applies across the age span, as it aims to restrict contact between children and vulnerable adults and those who might do them harm.

Safeguarding adults

The Centre for Public Scrutiny (2010) defined safeguarding adults as being

> *a range of activity aimed at upholding an adult's fundamental right to be safe at the same time as respecting people's rights to make choices. Safeguarding involves empowerment, protection and justice.*
>
> *(p. 4)*

This definition highlights the important balance between an adult's right to be safe and the adult's right to make choices. Legislation (HRA 1998, Equality Act 2010, MCA 2005) underpins the duty to empower people to make decisions and to be in control of their care and treatment. However, the balance between promoting both safety and independence can be delicate, as portrayed in Figure 10.1.

Faulkner and Sweeney (2011), from reviewing the literature, identified common interventions to prevent abuse as educating vulnerable adults

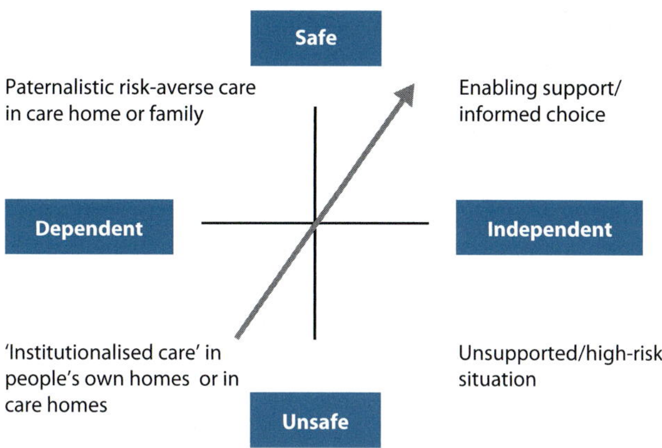

Figure 10.1 Independence and safety from abuse. 2008. (From Commission for Social Care Inspection. *Safeguarding Adults: A Study of the Effectiveness of Arrangements to Safeguard Adults from Abuse.* London: Commission for Social Care Inspection, p. 30.)

and staff so that they can recognise and respond to abuse; identifying people at risk of abuse; raising awareness and providing information, advice and advocacy; establishing policies, procedures, legislation and regulation; collaborating with other agencies; and a general emphasis on the promotion of empowerment and choice. Faulkner and Sweeney (2011) emphasison the importance of prevention in the context of person-centred support and personalisation, with individuals empowered to make choices and supported to manage risks. They provided a number of examples of initiatives to prevent abuse, such as educating people with learning disabilities who are at risk of being exploited and abused and projects involving community groups in prevention.

The DH and Home Office's (2000) document *No Secrets: Guidance on Developing and Implementing Multi-agency Policies and Procedures to Protect Vulnerable Adults from Abuse* set up a framework for adult safeguarding. This document will remain statutory guidance in England until at least 2014; legislation is under consideration (DH 2013). The *No Secrets* guidance required local authorities to establish multi-agency teams, with representatives from social services (the lead agency), the police, health authorities and NHS trusts. These 'safeguarding adults boards' have a remit to take protective measures by

1. Investigating allegations of abuse;
2. Assessing the extent to which a vulnerable adult requires support or protection; and, if necessary
3. Taking action against a perpetrator or a service or its management.

A review of *No Secrets* (DH 2009b) put more emphasis on prevention and the empowerment of individuals to maintain their own safety and achieve a balance between safeguarding and the independence associated with personalisation in adult social care. NHS trusts and healthcare practitioners must ensure that safeguarding adults is integrated with patient safety and clinical governance arrangements and with policies and procedures that ensure that safeguarding concerns are identified and managed safely (DH 2011). Further guidance from the DH (2013) built on previous DH publications and set out six safeguarding principles that provide a foundation for achieving good outcomes for patients (see Box 10.5).

Box 10.5

Safeguarding adults: principles*

Empowerment: There is presumption of person-led decisions and informed consent.
Prevention: It is better to take action before harm occurs.
Proportionality: Proportionate and least-intrusive response appropriate to the risk presented occurs.
Protection: There is support and representation for those in greatest need.
Partnership: Local solutions occur through services working with their communities. Communities have a part to play in preventing, detecting and reporting neglect and abuse.
Accountability: There is accountability and transparency in delivering safeguarding.

* From Department of Health (DH). 2013. *Statement of Government Policy on Adult Safeguarding.* London: Crown, p. 6.

Note that in Scotland, the Adult Support and Protection (Scotland) Act was passed in 2007. The act requires councils and a range of public bodies in Scotland to work together to support and protect adults who are unable to safeguard themselves, their property and their rights. In Northern Ireland, the Department of Health Social Services and Public Safety (DHSSPS) and the Department of Justice, supported by other government departments, are currently taking forward policy development in relation to safeguarding vulnerable adults in Northern Ireland.

The English government asserts that safeguarding is everybody's business, with communities having a role in preventing, identifying and reporting neglect and abuse, and measures in place locally to protect people least able to protect themselves (DH 2013). Multi-agency procedures apply if there is concern of neglect, harm or abuse to a patient who is defined as vulnerable (DH 2011). Safeguards against poor practice, harm and abuse must be an integral part of care and support services (DH 2013). The DH (2011) identified the key stages in safeguarding as follows:

1. Identify safeguarding concerns;
2. Make decisions–reasoned decisions about whether to refer through multi-agency procedures;
3. Provide multi-agency safeguarding responses by working in partnership to assess, investigate and develop a protection plan;
4. Evaluate outcomes and learning.

The concerns you may have will vary according to the degree of harm, the type of harm and the source of harm. However, reporting minor harms could lead to opportunities to prevent further harm.

In Box 10.4, although Nadia is apparently at risk of harm from her partner, one perspective is that she has the right to stay with him if that is her choice. However, her current mental health status makes her particularly vulnerable and could affect her decision-making. In addition, there are many complex factors that can prevent any adult who is suffering abuse from a partner, or another family member, from being able to take any action, but there are support services available (see http://www.nationaldomesticviolencehelpline.org.uk). At present, because she is in the mental health unit, Nadia is in a place of safety. However, Nadia's situation is further complicated by the concerns about her children, who remain with her partner. When responding to any concern about safeguarding adults, health workers must consider the implications for children, and the most urgent consideration in Nadia's case is that a person who is causing harm to an adult may also present a risk to children (DH 2011). When Nadia's discharge is being planned, other implications are that an adult's parenting capacity may be adversely affected by the stress of the abuse the adult is experiencing, and the choices that an adult makes about personal protection may adversely affect the adult's children (DH 2011).

From a more general mental health perspective on safeguarding, Whitelock (2009) asserted that the current adult safeguarding system is failing people with mental health problems and reported on research by Mind that demonstrated the urgent need for a prevention model of safeguarding, with service user involvement at its core and a rights-based approach. Whitelock (2009) argued that people feel disempowered by and frustrated with a paternalistic system that labels them vulnerable and fails to take account of their preferences in making decisions about their safety.

Abuse can occur in a range of environments, including NHS and voluntary organisations, private care homes and patients' personal residences, so nurses need to be aware of adults in their care who could be vulnerable to, and at risk of, abuse. Safeguarding of adults in institutions has increasingly emerged as institutional abuse has been recognised. The DH (2011) suggested that factors mitigating against institutional abuse are when there is strong leadership and a shared value base in which the patient is the primary concern; patients and carers are partners in their care; quality is prioritised and measured; staff are attuned to neglect, harm and abuse; there is a culture of improvement and learning, of openness and transparency; and all staff are listened to. It is also essential to have whistle-blowing policies in place alongside a culture that is open to scrutiny and in which all staff feel confident that they can raise concerns without fear of victimisation (DH 2011). Chapter 11 addresses whistle-blowing and associated issues in detail.

Heath and Phair (2010) proposed determinants of neglect that can be used to assist in decision-making processes; these include the effect on and consequences for the vulnerable person receiving care and whether the caregiver's actions were reasonable in the specific context. Thus, in relation to Mrs O'Connor (Box 10.3), an investigation into her care at the care home would need to consider the impact on her (of the pressure ulcer and her malnutrition) and what the care home staff did, for example, if they assessed her risk in relation to pressure ulcers and malnutrition and what steps they took to prevent these problems. It is important to determine whether the situation was the result of poor care or neglectful practice; the difference is determined by reviewing the effect of the omission on the patient (Heath and Phair 2009).

The Deprivation of Liberty Safeguards and restraint

Chapter 5 introduced you to the MCA (2005). The Deprivation of Liberty Safeguards (DOLS) are an amendment to the MCA that came into force in 2009, following a European Court of Human Rights ruling. (see http://www.equalityhumanrights.com/human-rights/our-human-rights-work/human-rights-inquiries/our-human-rights-inquiry/case-studies/the-bournewood-case/). The MCA DOLS apply to people in hospitals and care homes registered under the Care Standards Act of 2000, whether receiving the care through private arrangements or through public funding (DH 2009c). The DOLS provide legal protection for people in England and Wales who are over 18 years old and lack the capacity to consent to arrangements for their care and treatment. The DOLS are applicable when, after an independent assessment, deprivation of liberty (within the meaning of Article 5 of the HRA) may be in a person's best interests to protect the person from harm. The safeguards were designed to protect the interests of a vulnerable group of service users (e.g. persons with advanced dementia or persons with a profound learning disability). The aim is to make sure that a care home or hospital only deprives someone of liberty in a safe and correct way and only when it is in the best interests of the person and there is no other way to look after them. The DOLS aim to prevent arbitrary decisions that deprive vulnerable people of their liberty, provide safeguards for vulnerable people and provide them with the right to challenge unlawful detention. A review of the DOLS implementation by the House of Lords Select Committee and the Supreme Court in March 2014 led to further clarification of the 'acid test' for deprivation of liberty: that the person is subject to continuous supervision and control and is not free to leave, and the person lacks capacity to consent to these arrangements.

Examples of situations for which a DOLS application should be considered include whether to use restraint, including sedation, to admit a person who is resisting; if there is complete control over a person's care and movement for a significant period; when a person is prevented from leaving if the person makes a meaningful attempt to do so or if a request by carers to discharge the person to their care is denied; when a person is unable to maintain social contacts because of restrictions; or when a person loses autonomy because of continuous supervision and control. Watt and Brazier (2009) explained that any actions or restrictions imposed by healthcare professionals applying DOLS must operate within the five principles enshrined in the MCA in relation to a vulnerable adult, which are as follows:

1. A presumption of capacity;
2. The right for individuals to be supported in making decisions;
3. The right to make unwise decisions;
4. Best interests; and
5. Least-restrictive interventions.

Deprivation of liberty is only permitted to protect a person from harm; it should never be used for the convenience of others or as a form of punishment (Watt and Brazier 2009). The safeguards do not apply when someone is detained ('sectioned') under the Mental Health Act of 1983 (DH 2009c), so they would not apply to Nadia (Box 10.4) should she try to leave the unit.

To meet the safeguards, the role of best interest assessor (BIA) has been created. The BIA is a registered practitioner who has undergone additional training; the role involves promoting the rights, dignity and self-determination of individuals while being sensitive to their needs for personal respect, choice, and privacy (Watt and Brazier 2009).

There are two kinds of DOLS authorisations:

1) Standard authorisation is applied for before a deprivation of liberty occurs (e.g. part of a new care plan).

2) Urgent authorisation: can be made by managing authorities when there is an urgent need to deprive a person of their liberty but an application of a standard authorisation must be made at the same time to the supervisory body (DH 2009c).

The application is made to a local authority and is assessed by a BIA. DOLS applications are notifiable to the CQC and NHS England. The CQC (2011) provides useful guidance for care providers about the application of the DOLS.

In Mrs O'Connor's current state of acute delirium, she is unlikely to have the mental capacity to make the decision to go home, but an assessment of her capacity should be made rather than making assumptions, as a deprivation of liberty authorisation cannot be used if a person has the mental capacity to make decisions. As regards what is in her best interests, she might in fact recover better and her acute delirium could resolve more quickly if she was in a more familiar environment. However, as she is acutely unwell, there would need to be a suitable package of care in place, and the benefits and risks would need full discussion with Mrs O'Connor and her daughter. Watt and Brazier (2009) identified a key question when considering the use of DOLS: Is the level of risk sufficient to justify a step as serious as depriving a person of liberty?

Activity

Look back at Box 10.3, the scenario of Mrs O'Connor. What if Mrs O'Connor, during her state of acute delirium, was to express forcibly that she wanted to go home? Reflect on the following points:

1. Consider the five principles in the MCA. In particular, does Mrs O'Connor have the mental capacity to be able to make the decision to go home? Is it in Mrs O'Connor's best interests to go home? (She may mean her daughter's home rather than the care home.)
2. Would it be appropriate to apply the DOLS?
3. What other alternatives are there in handling this situation?

'Home' is somewhere most of us think of as a place of safety, comfort and security, and your reflection in the last activity might have prompted you to consider that Mrs O'Connor's stated wish to go home might be because she does not feel comfortable or safe in the ward environment. So, rather than consider DOLS, you might instead explore what Mrs O'Connor needs to make her feel more at ease, and a key point would be to work with her daughter on this. Could her daughter visit for longer–does the ward apply an open visiting policy? Is the ward team working in partnership with Mrs O'Connor and her daughter in a family-centred way? Chapters 7 and 8 explore these topics in detail. Are there familiar objects that Mrs O'Connor's daughter could bring in from home, like a framed photo, a cushion or blanket? Does Mrs O'Connor like music or books? Could you make these available to her? You could talk to Mrs O'Connor about things that are familiar to her and that she likes and enjoys. Remember that a key principle of DOLS is to provide care that is the least restricted possible; all options should be considered first.

The Alzheimer's Society (2013) provides a useful help sheet with specific reference to people with dementia and examples of when DOLS may or may not apply. The society suggests that it can be helpful to think of restrictions of a person's activity as being on a scale, from minimum restrictions at one end to the more extreme restrictions (deprivations of liberty) at the other end. In relation to people with learning disabilities, always consider their capacity to consent and their wishes (consult with their carer/next of kin/friends, as necessary). Consider whether an independent mental capacity advocate (IMCA) is needed and organise a best interests meeting. Other considerations include ensuring that there are reasonable adjustments and that the appropriate mode of communication is used to find out their wishes.

As regards use of restraints, the MCA (2005) allows the restraint of a person who lacks the capacity to make a particular decision in order to prevent them from being harmed. The restraint must not amount to the deprivation of liberty (in which case DOLS must be applied). The use of any form of restraint must always be a last resort, and all other options should be considered first. Types of restraint are as follows:

1. **Physical**: if a person is held by one or more persons in order to carry out medical care;
2. **Mechanical**: for example, application of bedrails to prevent a person getting out of bed or applying mittens to prevent a person pulling out an intravenous infusion;
3. **Chemical**: for example, sedation;

4. **Psychological**: for example, stopping someone from doing something by taking away something they need for mobility (e.g. spectacles or a walking aid).

Restraint must be in the best interests of the patient, for example, for essential treatment and care; it must be proportionate to the situation, that is, the least-restrictive option and the minimum to achieve the goal of safety. Therefore, although a soiled incontinence pad must be changed promptly to prevent skin damage and preserve dignity, if a person with advanced dementia initially refused to have an incontinence pad changed, rather than restraining the person to change it, you could try walking away and then returning after 5 minutes and using a different approach. Alternatively, you could find a colleague who has a particularly good relationship with the person to make the approach. Making a restraint decision requires careful assessment by an experienced individual and scrupulous documentation. Many organisations will have restraint policies and flowcharts to guide decision-making about, for example, use of bedrails or mittens, with specific documentation to record the assessment and documentation.

Activity

Find out about local processes and documentation for DOLS and restraints (e.g. use of bedrails or mittens) in your organisation:

- What documentation is used, and who must complete it?
- Who would ward staff contact if instigating DOLS was necessary?

Safeguarding children

The United Nations (1989) Convention on the Human Rights of the Child, which set out human rights for children, was ratified by the United Kingdom in 1991. Safeguarding children is a continually evolving area, as a result of national inquiries into children's deaths, reports of child trafficking and honour-based killings, as well as the emergence of new threats to children, such as cybersafety issues (Thornberry 2010). The DH (2013) asserted the following:

> *Ultimately, effective safeguarding of children can only be achieved by putting children at the centre of the system, and by every individual and agency playing their full part, working together to meet the needs of our most vulnerable children.*
>
> *(p. 9)*

The DH (2013) emphasised that safeguarding children, from pre-birth to 18 years, is 'everyone's responsibility' and that:

> *Everyone who works with children—including teachers, GPs [general practitioners], nurses, midwives, health visitors, early years professionals, youth workers, police, Accident and Emergency staff, paediatricians, voluntary and community workers and social workers—has a responsibility for keeping them safe.*
>
> *(p. 8)*

NICE (2009) identified that there is strong evidence of the harmful short- and long-term effects of child maltreatment on all aspects of the child's health, development and well-being. Furthermore, the effects of child maltreatment can last throughout adulthood and include anxiety, depression, substance misuse, and self-destructive, oppositional or anti-social behaviour (NICE 2009). The far-reaching effects also include difficulties with close relationships, sustaining employment and parenting capacity, while physical abuse may result in lifelong disability and harmful psychological consequences and may even be fatal (NICE 2009).

The 1989 Children Act, which was implemented in 1991, aimed to provide an effective legal framework for the safety and protection of children. All organisations offering services to children have a legal duty to safeguard children and promote well-being. The act enshrines five main principles: welfare, keeping the family together, non-intervention, avoidance of delay and unified laws and procedures (Griffith 2009). In 2004, through the Children Act, the government introduced Every Child Matters, which set out five statutory outcomes that are key for children and young people's well-being: be healthy, stay safe, enjoy and achieve, make a positive contribution and achieve economic well-being. This legislation applies in England and Wales.

In 2006, local safeguarding children boards (LSCBs) were established, replacing child protection committees. The LSCBs are statutory bodies and have more authority and a wider remit. Various policy and guidance documents have followed, and most recently, the English government (HM Government 2013) produced *Working Together to Safeguard Children: A Guide to Inter-agency Working to Safeguard and Promote the Welfare of Children*, which replaces the previous documents. The document defines safeguarding as being 'the action we take to promote the welfare of children and protect them from harm' (p. 7). HM Government (2013) further elaborated that safeguarding and promoting the welfare of children is

> *protecting children from maltreatment, preventing impairment of children's health or development, ensuring that children are growing up in*

> *circumstances consistent with the provision of safe and effective care, and taking action to enable all children to have the best chances.*
>
> (p. 7)

HM Government's (2013) definition of child protection is that it is

> *part of safeguarding and promoting welfare. This refers to the activity that is undertaken to protect specific children who are suffering, or are likely to suffer, significant harm.*
>
> (p. 85)

As you can see from this definition, safeguarding comprises a broader range of activities than child protection. The DH (2013) guidance is that all providers of NHS-funded health services should identify a named doctor and a named nurse (and a named midwife if the organisation provides maternity services) for safeguarding. An LSCB must be established for every local authority area; responsibilities include a range of roles and statutory functions, including developing local safeguarding policy and procedures and scrutinising local arrangements (DH 2013).

Box 10.6 outlines the attributes of an effective safeguarding system for children (DH 2013), which highlight the importance of all professionals in contact with children being alert to signs of abuse. Thus, the mental health team caring for Nadia (Box 10.4) have a responsibility to report concerns about her children. Local child safeguarding policies will set out who to contact, when and how. The attributes in Box 10.6 emphasise the importance of interprofessional and interagency communication.

Note that legislation varies between the UK countries, so ensure that you are familiar with the legislation in the country where you work. In Scotland, child protection is the responsibility of the Scottish government, and the legislative framework is the Children (Scotland) Act of 1995, which focusses on the needs of children and their families, defines parental responsibilities and rights relating to children, and presents the duties and powers available to public authorities to support children, and their families and to intervene when there are concerns about a child's welfare. The Protection of Children (Scotland) Act of 2003 presents measures to prevent unsuitable adults from working with children. In Northern Ireland, the Children (Northern Ireland) Order of 1995 was enabled in 1996, and it set out the authorities' responsibilities to provide services to children in need and their families, to provide for and support looked-after children, and to investigate children at risk and take appropriate action.

Box 10.6

Attributes of an effective safeguarding system for children*

- The child's needs are paramount, and the needs and wishes of each child, be they a baby or infant, or an older child, should be put first, so that every child receives the support they need before a problem escalates;
- All professionals who come into contact with children and families are alert to their needs and any risks of harm that individual abusers, or potential abusers, may pose to children;
- All professionals share appropriate information in a timely way and can discuss any concerns about an individual child with colleagues and local authority children's social care;
- High quality professionals are able to use their expert judgement to put the child's needs at the heart of the safeguarding system so that the right solution can be found for each individual child;
- All professionals contribute to whatever actions are needed to safeguard and promote a child's welfare and take part in regularly reviewing the outcomes for the child against specific plans and outcomes;
- Local Safeguarding Children Boards coordinate the work to safeguard children locally and monitor and challenge the effectiveness of local arrangements;
- When things go wrong Serious Case Reviews (SCRs) are published and transparent about any mistakes which were made so that lessons can be learnt; and
- Local areas innovate and changes are informed by evidence and examination of the data.

* From HM Government. 2013. *Working Together to Safeguard Children: A Guide to Inter-agency Working to Safeguard and Promote the Welfare of Children*. pp. 7–8. Available from: http://www.education.gov.uk/aboutdfe/statutory/g00213160/working-together-to-safeguard-children (accessed 14 October 2013).

Serious case reviews repeatedly raise poor interprofessional communication and a lack of interagency working as contributing factors to inadequate safeguarding of children (Banner 2012). NICE (2009) recommended effective communication between healthcare professionals and the child or young person and their families and carers that takes into account additional needs, such as physical, sensory or learning disabilities or any inability to speak or read English, and also considers cultural needs. As an example, the Coventry Safeguarding Children Board's (2013) serious review of the death of Daniel Pelka highlighted a wide range of communication issues; these included Daniel's perspective was not heard because he could not speak much English. Daniel's older sister, although a small child herself, was at times expected to interpret for her parents, who had briefed her to confirm their version of events. These factors, alongside many other issues, including a lack of interprofessional and interagency communication, contributed to the lack of recognition of Daniel's abuse.

The DH (2013) identified that no one professional can have a full picture of a child's needs and circumstances, and if children and families are to receive the right help at the right time, everyone who comes into contact with them has a role to play in identifying concerns, sharing information, writing accurate and comprehensive records, taking prompt action, and collaborating with other professionals. Practitioners should document observations, discussions, actions and decisions contemporaneously. As regards confidentiality of information shared, NICE (2009) guidance recommended that if healthcare professionals have concerns about sharing information with others, they should seek advice from named professionals for safeguarding children. If concerns are based on information given by a child, healthcare professionals should explain to the child when they are unable to maintain confidentiality, explore the child's concerns about sharing this information and reassure the child that they will continue to be kept informed about what is happening (NICE 2009). If health professionals are unsure what to share or with whom, they should discuss their concerns with a senior colleague or line manager (Thornberry 2010).

The DH (2013) emphasised that professionals should be alert to children needing early help, for example, children with disabilities; those with special educational needs; those with young carers; children who show signs of engaging in anti-social or criminal behaviour; if family circumstances present challenges for a child (e.g. substance abuse, adult mental health, domestic violence); or early signs of abuse or neglect exist. In the example of Nadia (Box 10.4), several of these points apply: the family circumstances (Nadia's mental health issues and the domestic violence) and early signs of neglect. The DH (2013) suggested an assessment framework for child safeguarding and promoting welfare (Figure 10.2). The framework takes a holistic approach, as it takes into account parental capacity, family and environmental factors, and the child's development needs.

Activity

Reflect on the scenario in Box 10.4. Which other professionals, apart from the mental health unit staff, could play a role in safeguarding Nadia's children?

You might have recognised that the children's teachers and other school staff have a key role. The DH (2013) identified a wide range

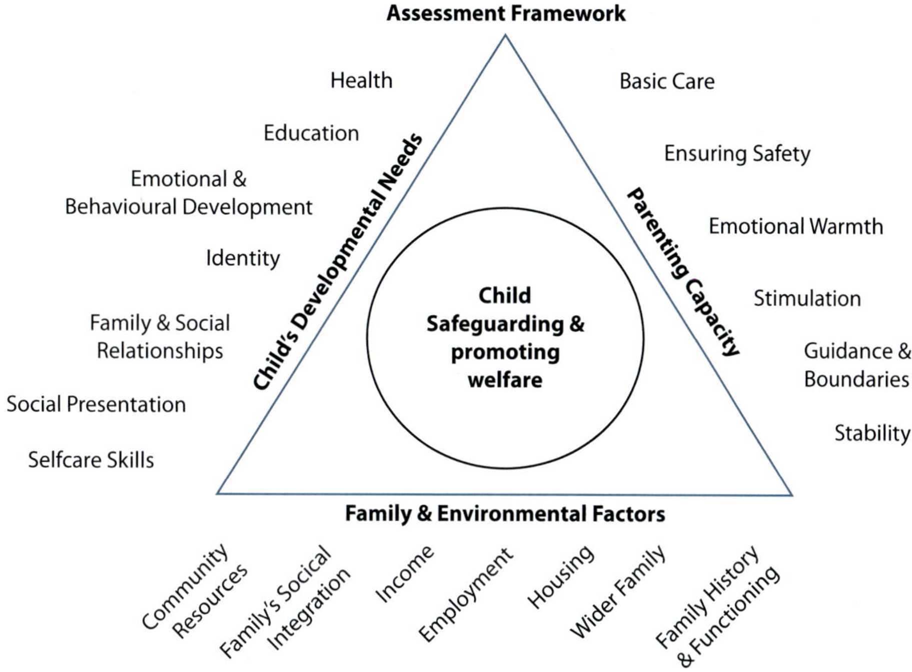

Figure 10.2 Assessment framework for safeguarding children and promoting welfare. (From: HM Government. 2013. *Working Together to Safeguard Children: A guide to inter-agency working to safeguard and promote the welfare of children*, p. 20. Available from: http://www.education.gov.uk/aboutdfe/statutory/g00213160/working-together-to-safeguard-children)

of health professionals who have a critical role to play in safeguarding and promoting the welfare of children, including GPs; primary care professionals; paediatricians; nurses; health visitors; midwives; school nurses; and those working in maternity, child and adolescent mental health, adult mental health, alcohol and drug services, unscheduled and emergency care settings and secondary and tertiary care. However, NICE (2009) acknowledged that healthcare professionals may encounter many different obstacles in the process of identifying maltreatment, including the following:

- They might be concerned about missing a treatable disorder.
- Healthcare professionals are used to working with parents and carers in the care of children and fear losing a positive relationship with a family already under their care.
- There is the discomfort of disbelieving, thinking ill of, suspecting or wrongly blaming a parent or carer.

- The professionals have divided duties to adult and child patients and a concern about breaching confidentiality.
- They have an understanding of the reasons why the maltreatment might have occurred and that there was no intention to harm the child.
- They fear losing control over the child protection process and have doubts about its benefits.
- Stress is a factor.
- They have concerns for personal safety.
- There is a fear of complaints.

Thornberry (2010) also identified the 'start again syndrome', by which practitioners often ignored or minimized previous concerns, and new events, such as the birth of a baby were seen as a fresh start for a family.

Chapter summary

Nurses in most settings work with people who are vulnerable to harm; this chapter focussed particularly on people with learning disabilities, children, older people and people with mental health issues. However, anyone of any age can be vulnerable to harm, and nurses must be alert and vigilant in identifying risks and any signs of abuse, not only in people they are caring for but also other family members. We must also ensure that safeguarding takes place in the context of empowering individuals in our society to protect themselves and make their own choices whenever possible. There have been many new policies and legislation relevant to safeguarding in recent years, and it is important to keep up to date with the developments in this field, especially in the country where you are working. It is vital that you are familiar with local policies and procedures within your organisation and that you attend the mandatory training relating to this topic. Above all, remember that safeguarding adults and children is everyone's business, and effective interprofessional and interagency communication and collaboration are vital.

Acknowledgement

We are grateful to Vicki Leah, Consultant Nurse for Older People, University College London Hospitals, for critically reviewing this chapter.

Useful resources

Action for Advocacy. 2007. Good practice in advocacy publication list. http://www.actionforadvocacy.org.uk/articleServlet?action=display&article=774&articletype=28&page=2.

Action on Elder Abuse. Home page. http://www.elderabuse.org.uk/.

Age UK. Home page. http://www.ageuk.org.uk/.

Barnardo's. Home page. http://www.barnardos.org.uk.

Care Quality Commission. Home page. http://www.cqc.org.uk/.

Mencap. Home page. http://www.mencap.org.uk/.

National Society for the Prevention of Cruelty to Children (NSPCC). Home page. http://www.nspcc.org.uk/.

Nursing and Midwifery Council (NMC). 2013. *Introduction to Safeguarding Adults*. http://www.nmc-uk.org/Nurses-and-midwives/Regulation-in-practice/Safeguarding-New/Introduction-to-safeguarding-adults/.

Nursing and Midwifery Council (NMC). n.d. *Safeguarding Adults | An Introduction* (series of films). http://www.nmc-uk.org/Nurses-and-midwives/safeguarding-film-one-an-introduction/.

Safe: The Safe Network. 2011. *Why Does Safeguarding Matter and Why Does It Matter to My Organisation?* http://www.safenetwork.org.uk/getting_started/Pages/Why_does_safeguarding_matter.aspx.

Social Care Institute for Excellence. n.d. *Adult Safeguarding*. http://www.scie.org.uk/adults/safeguarding/.

Social Care Institute for Excellence. n.d. List of safeguarding adults videos on Social Care TV. http://www.scie.org.uk/socialcaretv/topic.asp?t=safeguardingadults.

Social Care Institute for Excellence. n.d. List of safeguarding children videos on Social Care TV. http://www.scie.org.uk/socialcaretv/topic.asp?t=safeguardingchildren.

Welsh Government. Violence against Women and Domestic Abuse. http://wales.gov.uk/topics/people-and-communities/safety/domestic-abuse/?lang=en.

Women's Aid. Home page. http://www.womensaid.org.uk/.

Women's Aid and Refuge 24-Hour National Domestic Violence Freephone Helpline. 2012. Home page. http://www.nationaldomesticviolencehelpline.org.uk/

References

Action on Elder Abuse (AEA). 2012. *What Is Elder Abuse?* Available from: http://www.elderabuse.org.uk/Mainpages/Abuse/abuse.html (accessed 27 September 2013).

Adult Support and Protection (Scotland) Act. 2007. Available from http://www.legislation.gov.uk/asp/2007/10/contents (accessed 23 April 2014).

Age UK. 2012. *Safeguarding Older People from Abuse*. Fact sheet 78. Available from: http://www.ageuk.org.uk/brandpartnerglobal/eastlondonvpp/documents/fs78_safeguarding_older_people_from_abuse_fcs.pdf (accessed 5 October 2013).

Alzheimer's Society. 2013. *Deprivation of Liberty Safeguards*. Available from: http://www.alzheimers.org.uk/site/scripts/download_info.php?fileID=1830 (accessed 1 December 2013).

Banner, J. 2012. Addressing safeguarding concerns through better communication. *Nursing Management* 19(2): 28–31.

British Geriatrics Society. 2011. *Joint Working Party Inquiry into the Quality of Healthcare Support for Older People in Care Homes: A Call for Leadership, Partnership and Quality Improvement*. London: British Geriatrics Society.

Brocklehurst, H., Laurenson, M. 2008. A concept analysis examining the vulnerability of older people. *British Journal of Nursing* 17(21): 1354–1357.

Care Quality Commission (CQC). 2011. *The Mental Capacity Act 2005 Deprivation of Liberty Safeguards: Guidance for Providers*. Available from: http://www.cqc.org.uk/sites/default/files/media/documents/rp_poc1b2b_100564_20111223_v4_00_guidance_for_providers_mca_dols_for_external_publication.pdf (accessed 14 October 2013).

Care Quality Commission (CQC). 2013a. *Our Safeguarding Protocol: The Care Quality Commission's Responsibility and Commitment to Safeguarding*. Available from: http://www.cqc.org.uk/sites/default/files/media/documents/20130123_800693_v2_00_cqc_safeguarding_protocol.pdf (accessed 14 October 2013).

Care Quality Commission (CQC). 2013b. *Time to Listen in Care Homes: Dignity and Nutrition Inspection Programme 2012*. Available from: http://www.cqc.org.uk/sites/default/files/media/documents/time_to_listen_-_care_homes_main_report_tag.pdf (accessed 4 October 2013).

Care Quality Commission (CQC). 2013c. *Time to Listen in Hospitals: Dignity and Nutrition Inspection Programme 2012*. Available from: http://www.cqc.org.uk/public/publications/themed-inspections/dignity-and-nutrition-older-people/dignity-and-nutrition-nhs (accessed 4 October 2013).

Care Standards Act. 2000. Available from: http://www.legislation.gov.uk/ukpga/2000/14/contents (accessed 23 April 2014).

Centre for Public Scrutiny, Improvement and Development Agency. 2010. *Adult Safeguarding Scrutiny Guide*. London: Improvement and Development Agency.

Children Act. 1989. Available from: http://www.legislation.gov.uk/ukpga/1989/41/contents (accessed 23 April 2014).

Children Act. 2004. Available from: http://www.legislation.gov.uk/ukpga/2004/31/contents (accessed 23 April 2014).

Children (Scotland) Act. 1995. Available from: http://www.legislation.gov.uk/ukpga/1995/36/contents (accessed 23 April 2014).

Commission for Social Care Inspection. 2008. *Safeguarding Adults: A Study of the Effectiveness of Arrangements to Safeguard Adults from Abuse*. London: Commission for Social Care Inspection.

Cornwall Adult Protection Committee. 2007. *The Murder of Stephen Hoskin: A Serious Case Review: Executive Summary*. Available from: http://www.pkc.gov.uk/CHttpHandler.ashx?id=14720&p=0 (accessed 14 October 2013).

Coventry Safeguarding Children Board. 2013. *Serious Case Review*: Re Daniel Pelka. Available from: http://www.coventrylscb.org.uk/files/SCR/FINAL%20Overview%20Report%20%20DP%20130913%20Publication%20version.pdf (accessed 1 January 2014).

Cowley, J., Lee, S. 2011. Safeguarding people's rights under the Mental Capacity Act. *Nursing Older People* 23(1): 19–23.

de Chesnay, M., Robinson-Dooley, V. 2012. Vulnerable populations, vulnerable people. In de Chesnay, M., and Anderson, B.A. (eds.), *Caring for the Vulnerable*. 3rd ed. Burlington, MA: Jones and Bartlett Learning, 3–16.

Department of Health (DH). 2009a. *Valuing People Now*. London: DH.

Department of Health (DH). 2009b. *Safeguarding Adults: Report on the Consultation on the Review of No Secrets*. London: DH.

Department of Health (DH). 2009c. *Deprivation of Liberty Safeguards: A Guide for Hospitals and Care Homes*. Gateway reference 11229. London: DH.

Department of Health (DH). 2010. *Prioritising Need in the Context of Putting People First: A Whole System Approach to Eligibility for Social Care. Guidance on Eligibility Criteria for Adult Social Care, England 2010*. Gateway reference 13729. London: DH.

Department of Health (DH). 2011. *Safeguarding Adults: The Role of Healthcare Practitioners*. Gateway reference 15738. London: DH.

Department of Health (DH). 2012. *Transforming Care: A National Response to Winterbourne View Hospital: Department of Health Review: Final Report* Gateway reference 18348. Available from: https://www.gov.uk/government/publications/winterbourne-view-hospital-department-of-health-review-and-response (accessed 22 June 2013).

Department of Health (DH). 2013. *Statement of Government Policy on Adult Safeguarding*. London: Crown.

Department of Health (DH) and Home Office. 2000. *No Secrets: Guidance on Developing and Implementing Multi-Agency Policies and Procedures to Protect Vulnerable Adults from Abuse.* London: DH.

Dorsen, C. 2010. Vulnerability in homeless adolescents: Concept analysis. *Journal of Advanced Nursing* 66(12): 2819–2827.

Equality Act. 2010. Available from: http://www.legislation.gov.uk/ukpga/2010/15/contents (accessed 23 April 2014).

Faulkner, A., Sweeney, A. 2011. *Prevention in Adult Safeguarding: A Review of the Literature.* London: Social Care Institute for Excellence.

Flaskerud, J., Winslow, B.J. 1998. Conceptualizing vulnerable population's health-related research. *Nursing Research* 47(2): 69–78.

Fyson, R., Kitson, D. 2010. Human rights and social wrongs: Issues in safeguarding adults with learning disabilities. *Practice* 22(5): 309–320.

Griffith, R. 2009. Safeguarding Children: Key concepts and principles. *British Journal of School Nursing* 4(7): 335–340.

Heath, H., Phair, L. 2009. The concept of frailty and its significance in the consequences of care or neglect for older people: An analysis. *International Journal of Older People Nursing* 4(2): 120–131.

Heath, H., Phair, L. 2010. Neglect of older people in formal care settings part one: New perspectives on definition and the nursing contribution to multi-agency safeguarding work. *Journal of Adult Protection* 12(3): 5–13.

Health Service Ombudsman. 2011. *Care and Compassion? Report of the Health Service Ombudsman on Ten Investigations into NHS Care of Older People.* Available from: http://www.ombudsman.org.uk/care-and-compassion/home (accessed 16 October 2013).

Heslop, P., Blair, P., Fleming, P., Hoghton, M., Marriott, A., Russ, L. 2013. Confidential Inquiry into Premature Deaths of People with Learning Disabilities (CIPOLD). Available from: http://www.bristol.ac.uk/cipold/fullfinalreport.pdf (accessed 14 October 2013).

HM Government. 2013. Working Together to Safeguard Children: A Guide to Inter-agency Working to Safeguard and Promote the Welfare of Children. Available from: http://www.education.gov.uk/aboutdfe/statutory/g00213160/working-together-to-safeguard-children (accessed 14 October 2013).

House of Lords/House of Commons. 2007. *Joint Committee On Human Rights—The Human Rights of Older People in Healthcare*. Eighteenth Report. Available from: http://www.publications.parliament.uk/pa/jt200607/jtselect/jtrights/156/15602.htm (accessed 2 July 2012).

Human Rights Act. 1998. Available from: http://www.legislation.gov.uk/ukpga/1998/42/contents (accessed 23 April 2014).

Jenkins, R., Davies, R. 2011. Safeguarding people with learning disabilities. *Learning Disability Practice* 14(1): 32–39.

Law Commission. 2011. *Adult Social Care Consultation Analysis.* Consultation Paper No. 192 (Consultation Analysis). London: Law Commission.

Mencap. 2004. *Treat Me Right! Better Healthcare for People with a Learning Disability*. London: Mencap.

Mencap. 2007. *Death by Indifference: Following up the Treat Me Right!* London: Mencap.

Mencap. 2012. *Death by Indifference: 74 Deaths and Counting: A Progress Report 5 Years On.* London: Mencap.

Mental Capacity Act. 2005. Available from: http://www.legislation.gov.uk/ukpga/2005/9/contents (accessed 23 April 2014).

Mercer, D. 2013. Hospital workers jailed for abusing female patients on Whipps Cross geriatric ward. *The Independent*. Available from: http://www.independent.co.uk/life-style/health-and-families/health-news/hospital-workers-jailed-for-abusing-female-patients-on-whipps-cross-geriatric-ward-8782397.html (accessed 5 October 2013).

National Institute for Health and Clinical Excellence (NICE). 2009. *When to Suspect Child Maltreatment*. Clinical guideline 89. Available from: http://guidance.nice.org.uk/CG89 (accessed 16 October 2013).

National Institute for Health and Clinical Excellence (NICE). 2012. *Social and Emotional Wellbeing: Early Years*. Public health guidance 40. Available from: http://publications.nice.org.uk/social-and-emotional-wellbeing-early-years-ph40/recommendations#home-visiting-early-education-and-childcare (accessed 16 October 2013).

Northway, R. 2002. The nature of vulnerability. *Learning Disability Practice* 5(6): 26.

Nursing and Midwifery Council (NMC). 2008. *The Code: Standards of Conduct, Performance and Ethics for Nurses and Midwives.* London: NMC.

O'Keeffe, M., Hills, A., Doyle, M., et al. 2007. *UK Study of Abuse and Neglect of Older People: Prevalence Survey Report.* Completed for Comic Relief and the Department of Health. London: National Centre for Social Research.

Protection of Children (Scotland) Act. 2003. Available from: http://www.legislation.gov.uk/asp/2003/5 (accessed 23 April 2014).

Perry, J. 2004. Hate crime against people with learning difficulties: The role of the Crime and Disorder Act and No Secrets in identification and prevention. *Journal of Adult Protection* 6(1): 27–34.

Phair, L., Heath, H. 2012. Safeguarding vulnerable older people in hospital. *Nursing Standard* 27(4): 50–55.

Royal College of Nursing (RCN). 2007. *Safeguarding Children and Young People: Every Nurse's Responsibility: Guidance for Nursing Staff.* London: RCN.

Royal College of Nursing (RCN). 2010. *Mental Health Nursing of People with Learning Disabilities: RCN Guidance.* London: RCN.

Safeguarding Vulnerable Groups Act. 2006. Available from: http://www.legislation.gov.uk/ukpga/2006/47/contents (accessed 23 April 2014).

Schröder-Butterfill, E., Marianti, R. 2006. A framework for understanding old age vulnerabilities. *Ageing and Society* 26(1): 9–35.

Scottish Human Rights Commission (SHRC). 2011. *Evaluation of Care about Rights*. Phase 2: Report to the Scottish Human Rights Commission. October 2011. Available from: http://www.scottishhumanrights.com/application/resources/documents/CaRfullevaluationfinalOct2011.pdf (accessed 1 December 2013).

Straughair, C. 2011. Safeguarding vulnerable adults: The role of the registered nurse. *Nursing Standard* 25(45): 49–56.

Tadd, W., Hillman, A., Calnan, S., et al. 2011. *Dignity in Practice: An Exploration of the Care of Older Adults in Acute NHS Trusts.* NIHR Service Delivery and Organisation Programme. Available from: http://www.bgs.org.uk/pdf_cms/reference/Tadd_Dignity_in_Practice.pdf (accessed 23 April 2014).

Tang, K.L., Lee, J.J. 2006. Global social justice for older people: The case for an international convention on the rights of older people. *British Journal of Social Work* 36(7): 1135–1150.

The Children (Northern Ireland) Order. 1995. Available from: http://www.legislation.gov.uk/nisi/1995/755/contents/made (accessed 23 April 2014).

Thornberry, M. 2010. Safeguarding children: An essential guide. *Practice Nursing* 21(4):179–183.

United Nations. 1948. *Universal Declaration of Human Rights*. Available from: http://www.un.org/en/documents/udhr/ (accessed 16 October 2013).

United Nations. 1989. *Convention on the Human Rights of the Child*. Available from: http://www.ohchr.org/EN/ProfessionalInterest/Pages/CRC.aspx (accessed 16 October 2013).

United Nations. 1991. *Implementation of the International Plan of Action on Ageing and Related Activities.* Available from: http://www.un.org/documents/ga/res/46/a46r091.htm (accessed 22 November 2013).

Watt, G., Brazier, L. 2009. Safeguarding vulnerable adults' liberty: Creating a new role. *Learning Disability Practice* 12(8): 18–21.

Whitelock, A. 2009. Safeguarding in mental health: Towards a rights-based approach. *Journal of Adult Protection* 11(4): 30–42.

11

Challenging poor practice and raising concerns

Introduction

You will have seen examples in Chapter 3 and in other chapters of this book that there are times when care is below the standard expected. When reviewing the professional code in Chapter 2 and public expectations of nurses in Chapter 3, you will have read about the requirement to uphold the standards of the nursing profession and to safeguard vulnerable people in your care, as discussed at length in Chapter 10. One question that is often asked is why nurses do not, or do little to, report concerns about poor care. This chapter focusses on the importance of challenging poor practice as a student and registered nurse and the need to challenge and report discrimination, poor standards of care and poor working practices. Whistle-blowing is explored in the light of legal, ethical and professional duties to report. The skills and courage required of nurses to communicate concerns, deal with confidentiality dilemmas and report colleagues are all addressed.

Learning outcomes

By the end of this chapter, you will be able to

- Discuss the concept of whistle-blowing, and the duty to report concerns, within legal, ethical and professional contexts;
- Appreciate the courage and skills required to challenge poor practice and raise concerns;
- Reflect on your own skills and confidence that will ensure that you can recognise, raise and report concerns.

Whistle-blowing

The term *whistle-blowing* can have negative connotations as it has often been used when describing someone who has gone outside an organisation to report concerns to the press. Whistle-blowing has been defined as

> *the disclosure by organisation members (former or current) of illegal, immoral, or illegitimate practices under the control of their employers, to persons or organizations that may be able to effect action.*
>
> *(Near & Miceli 1985, p. 4)*

Ahern and McDonald (2002) took this definition further by suggesting that a whistle-blower is

> *someone who identifies an incompetent, unethical or illegal situation in the workplace and reports it to someone who has the power to stop the wrong.*
>
> *(p. 303)*

Firtko and Jackson (2005) added a layer to this definition by suggesting that whistle-blowing occurs when an employee reports something that would normally be viewed as confidential to an agency outside their organisation.

Griffith and Tengnah (2012) suggested that public interest disclosure or whistle-blowing occurs when a worker discloses information about poor practice at work. Here, the words *public interest* are key and appear in the definition provided by GOV.UK (2013), which suggests that whistle-blowing is 'making a disclosure in the public interest' and occurs when an employee reports practice that is illegal or practice that is neglectful. This could include the 'qualifying disclosures' (GOV.UK 2013) of breach of health and safety law (in nursing, this could relate to the environment or shortage of necessary equipment, for example) or a criminal offence (assault, battery or theft, for example), that the organisation is flouting the law, or a wrongdoing has been covered up (GOV.UK 2013).

Near and Miceli (1985) suggested that there are four components to whistle-blowing: the whistle-blower, the act of whistle-blowing (or complaint), the person or organisation to whom the complaint is made, and the organisation or person against which the complaint is made. They also suggested that there are four characteristics of whistle-blowers: The whistle-blower must have at some stage been employed by the organisation within which the transgression occurred; the whistle-blower is an individual who does not have the authority to influence the behaviour within the organisation; there is an assumption that the whistle-blower will remain anonymous; and the whistle-blower occupies a role that requires action on his or her concerns (Near and Miceli 1985).

Regardless of the definition of whistle-blowing, it is clear that the reporting of concerns should be in the interest of the public, the people to whom you are providing care. The disclosure should not be made to benefit you as an individual in your professional role or for your own personal financial gain. It is suggested here that 'raising concerns' is a more fitting terminology as it removes the negative connotations associated with the word *whistle-blowing*.

Why do nurses raise concerns?

Ahern and McDonald (2002) found that those who do report concerns about misconduct believe first and foremost in patient advocacy, whereas nurses who do not raise concerns believe in the traditional role of nursing. Jackson et al. (2011) further suggested that those nurses who report concerns are acting in accordance with their duty of care. This could suggest that those nurses who do not raise concerns are in fact neglecting their duty of care.

Berry (2004) suggested that reporting concerns enables nurses to maintain the ethics of truth telling, the promotion of justice and the redressing of wrong. Firtko and Jackson (2005) further posited that concerns are reported to improve quality and maintain high standards in practice, and this may take the form of completing incident forms or informing line managers or other appropriate staff of concerns.

Therefore, nurses will raise concerns because they are committed to promoting high standards of care and protecting those in their care. This commitment would lead them to raise concerns despite any potential risk to themselves. This could suggest that these nurses have a role morality which is the work nurses do to meet care needs and this includes reporting concerns about standards of care (Hanna 2004). It can also be suggested that these nurses have a high level of moral integrity. Consider the scenario presented in Box 11.1.

Box 11.1

Practice scenario: reporting concerns about a colleague's competence

You are working in the community and have been assessed as competent to carry out a follow-up visit to Paul. Paul's carer, Jane, is always present when he is visited by the nurse. Jane mentions that Lisa, who was supposed to visit yesterday, did not arrive. Jane says that when Lisa does visit she is disorganised, is flippant with her remarks to Paul and does not seem to care. Jane feels that Paul is being put at risk by Lisa's practice. You have heard of other comments made in relation to Lisa's competence.

Consider your principles and values relating to this situation from a consequentialist stance and a deontological stance. Question whether or not you would report and consider the rationale for your decision.

If you do raise a concern, you may do so using an ethical framework. Wilmot (2000) suggested that if you are reporting concerns in order to change or improve a situation, then you would be adopting a consequentialist position (being concerned with consequences and outcomes, doing what is right, greatest good utilitarian principle, the ends justifying the means), but if you see your actions to report as your duty to do so, you are probably adopting a deontological stance (obligation, doing what is right regardless of the consequences). For a more detailed explanation of consequentialism and deontology, see Chapter 4.

Courage to communicate concerns

Lachman (2007) described moral courage as the individual ability and capacity to overcome fear and openly support one's core values. Courage is necessary to deal with everyday fears, and to be morally responsible for care requires the ability to recognise and respond to poor practice (LaSala and Bjarnason 2010). Therefore, courage is a really important virtue when it comes to communicating concerns. Lindh et al. (2010) suggested that nurses must have the courage to 'recognise what is', have insight into 'what could be' and act on 'what ought to be' (p. 564). To demonstrate courage, healthcare professionals must put their patients' needs before any threat to themselves (LaSala and Bjarnason 2010); they must have the courage to stand up for what they think is right despite the consequences to them personally or professionally, therefore remaining true to their professional values and beliefs (Laabs 2011).

Having the courage to act has a positive impact on care standards. It requires healthcare professionals to stand firm in their beliefs of what is right (Lindh et al. 2009). This does, however, require organisations to empower staff and provide an environment that supports ethical practice (Fry et al. 2002). Courage is important in the nursing profession, especially when the competence of others needs to be challenged (Epstein and Hamric 2009) and there is a need to do something about bad practice (Day 2007).

Activity

Read the report *To Whistleblow Is Like a Death Sentence: Five People Who Risked Everything to Speak Out* (C. Cooper. March 23, 2013. http://www.independent.co.uk/news/people/profiles/to-whistleblow-is-like-a-death-sentence-five-people-who-risked-everything-to-speak-out-8542421.html) and reflect on how the people in the report felt about their experience.

The personal risk of not raising a concern: moral distress and residue

On identifying a concern about standards of care or professional practice, because you recognise a conflict with your values and beliefs, you may feel frustrated, angry or anxious (Jameton 1984). The Royal College of Nursing

(RCN) (2011) identified that 80 per cent of nurses leave work feeling some level of distress because they were unable to provide the care they knew was right. In nursing practice, the environment influences ethical standards, as does support from colleagues and the norms of practice, and if there is a struggle to maintain integrity this can lead to moral distress (Kelly 1996, 1998).

Moral distress can be the result of you knowing what is the right thing to do but being unable to do anything about it because of organisational constraints, and reactive moral distress is the distress nurses experience when they do not do anything to address or rectify poor standards (Jameton 1984). It could also arise because of a conflict between your commitment to the organisation and your commitment to those in your care (Corley et al. 2005). If your core values are challenged and infringed, this can also lead to moral distress, which can have a really negative impact on you (Epstein and Hamric 2009).

Webster and Baylis (2000) made further links between what an individual actually does and what transpires (i.e. the consequences); therefore, if a nurse decides not to pursue the right course of action to rectify his or her concerns, the nurse will experience a continued feeling of moral distress. The act of doing nothing may not always be a deliberate or malicious choice. There might be an error of judgement on the nurse's part, because of a personal failing or because of circumstances out of the nurse's control (Webster and Baylis 2000).

Severe signs of moral distress, if ignored and left unresolved, result in moral residue (Edmonson 2010). Webster and Baylis (2000) suggested that if you have compromised yourself or allowed your integrity to be compromised by others, then you will experience moral residue by carrying this distress with you. They described two causes of moral distress:

1. The realisation of an error, and,
2. An incremental loss of commitment to previously held values for reasons of self-interest (self-protection or self-promotion). (p. 218).

Moral residue can lead to further mistakes in the future because of the loss of commitment to professional values and resulting compromised integrity (Webster and Baylis 2000). However, the converse may apply, with some individuals, who may take a different course of action in the future because they have recognised why this residue exists, and their moral values and commitment have been clarified and reinforced (Webster and Baylis 2000).

Review Box 11.2 and consider the scenario from two different courses of action: the first being the decision to report your concerns, and the second being where you decide to do nothing about the situation.

Box 11.2

Practice scenario: reporting concerns about inpatient acute care

You are working in an acute inpatient environment; you notice that the nurses treat people in need of nursing care differently to what you have observed previously. The nurses are quite rough, and they rush around doing everything quickly, often not delivering dignified care. The people receiving this care are confused and do not understand what is being 'done' to them because the care is not explained; they are therefore becoming distressed. The nurses say that they are short staffed, but that this is normal, so they just get on with it. They do not have the time to provide appropriate levels of care.

You are considering whether to report these concerns. Reflect on your decision in relation to your personal and professional values and beliefs and the consequences of your actions.

If you did nothing about the situation discussed in Box 11.2, then the poor care would continue. Should you accept that this is in fact normal practice? If you do nothing, you may find that you are also held accountable for the failings in the care. You could raise these concerns with your mentor, the nurse in charge, the matron or one of your lecturers. If you do not feel anything is changing, you will probably find that most senior nurses or directors of nursing would be keen to hear your concerns directly. Some National Health Service (NHS) trusts organise forums at which senior staff meet with students to hear their perspectives about care in the trust.

Raising a concern

As highlighted in the previous material, raising a concern in practice can be stressful. What then should you do and how should you go about it? Berry (2004) suggested that whilst there may be a need to report concerns both internal to and external of an organisation, there is greater benefit to an organisation when employees report internally because this facilitates earlier investigation and enables organisations to be more proactive in the management of misconduct. Firtko and Jackson (2005) further advocated internal reporting that occurs as a result of specific guidelines within an organisation. This could be a nurse reporting a concern because a colleague has not practised in accordance with approved policies or procedures. So, do first consider who you can go to internally within the organisation to discuss your concerns.

Often, a concern can arise because you observe care that conflicts with your own values and beliefs about what good standards of care are. If a person in your care has obviously been physically assaulted or abused deliberately (i.e. hit), it may be easier to do something about it, and in this case you should tell someone immediately. According to the Nursing and Midwifery Council (NMC) (2013, p. 2):

> *Abuse may be deliberate or the result of negligence or ignorance, and includes physical, psychological or sexual abuse, financial or material abuse, neglect, failure to act or institutional abuse.*

If you do observe such abuse, it will be necessary to report this immediately through your organisation's safeguarding process. If you do not report such abuse, you could potentially be held as responsible for the outcomes of that abuse (including neglect and omissions of care) as the person who carried out that abuse. You must always prioritise the needs and safety of the people in your care.

The NMC (2013), Care Quality Commission (CQC) (2012) and the RCN (2013) have produced guidance to support nurses and midwives, including nursing and midwifery students, who wish to raise concerns. The NMC (2013) guidance has been written to reflect the Code (NMC 2008) and is therefore underpinned by professional expectations. All sets of guidance should be read and used in conjunction with your organisation's policy for raising concerns or whistle-blowing.

Activity

Look for the policy or process for raising a concern within your university and within your practice area.

- What are the key steps within these processes? Are they similar?
- Would you feel confident raising a concern using these processes?
- Compare these policies to the guidance produced by the NMC (2013), CQC (2012), and RCN (2013).

As a student nurse, the NMC (2009) states that if you believe that you, a colleague or anyone else is putting someone at risk of harm, you should immediately inform your mentor or lecturer. In addition, if someone in your care has suffered harm you must inform the professional best qualified to help that person. Equally, if anyone in your care is dissatisfied with the care they receive or how they have been treated, you must inform your mentor or lecturer (NMC 2009). If, as a registered nurse, you fail to report concerns, this may bring your fitness to practise into question and put your registration at risk (NMC 2013).

The NMC (2013) suggests that if you have a concern as a student, ideally, you should adhere to the employer's policy for raising concerns or whistle-blowing. However, under the NMC (2009) guide for students, they suggest you should do the following:

- Inform your mentor, tutor or lecturer immediately if you believe that you, a colleague or anyone else may be putting someone at risk of harm.
- Seek help immediately from an appropriately qualified professional if someone for whom you are providing care has suffered harm for any reason.
- Seek help from your mentor, tutor or lecturer if people indicate that they are unhappy about their care or treatment.

If you have observed poor practice or the mistreatment of someone in your care, consider the seven points in Box 11.3 to guide you in making your judgement and raising your concern.

Box 11.3

Seven points to consider when raising a concern

1. Ask yourself whether the practice you are witnessing is illegal, unprofessional, or immoral; breaches policies or processes; or causes harm to the person receiving the care.
2. If you are unsure about what you have witnessed or experienced, seek advice and support from a colleague, mentor, fellow student, or university lecturer or, if you feel unable to do so, an outside agency such as the RCN or PCAW (Public Concern at Work).
3. Ensure that you have clear facts about what you have witnessed or experienced and that you have written this down so that you do not forget anything. This should include names of those involved, times, dates, observations and any discussions.
4. Weigh the consequences for you reporting and not reporting for the following:
   a. **You** (if you either raise a concern or do nothing about your concern)
   b. **The organisation** (if you either raise a concern or do nothing about your concern)
   c. **Your colleagues** (if you either raise a concern or do nothing about your concern)
   d. **The person receiving the care** (if you either raise a concern or do nothing about your concern)
5. Is the person or organisation you are reporting to best placed to address your concern?
6. Is there any other way you could address your concern?
7. If you decide to raise a concern, you should be able to justify your concern based on procedural, ethical, legal or professional grounds, and you must take responsibility for your decision.

Protection for employees under law

Protection for the employee who wishes to raise a concern or whistle-blow is now embedded in the NHS Constitution (Department of Health 2013). It is now clear that all those employees working in the NHS have a duty to report concerns about poor practice as soon as possible. In addition, NHS organisations must ensure concerns are taken seriously and are investigated fully, supporting staff throughout these investigations. However, issues of confidentiality are often unclear. In the context of raising concerns, Jackson et al. (2011) suggested that healthcare organisations often withhold information intentionally, and in these circumstances, confidentiality is used to protect healthcare organisations from public inquiry. However, the notion of enforced confidentiality is also raised if nurses who raise concerns may be forced to remain silent and not share their concerns with colleagues (Jackson et al. 2011). This may be another reason why nurses are reluctant to raise concerns. Confidentiality should be used to protect the individual raising the concern, and Moore and McAuliffe (2010) called for the need to address concerns about confidentiality because individuals are fearful of their colleagues seeing a written statement and judging or blaming them.

The culture within an organisation also has a significant impact on how employees are protected when trying to raise a concern. Berry (2004) presented seven dimensions of organisational culture, which can either enable or get in the way of employees reporting concerns:

1. **Vigilance:** Individuals are required to be aware of expected values and standards and be attentive to breaches of these standards.
2. **Engagement:** Individuals need to be committed to high ethical standards and be cognisant of what they are willing to do for their organisation.
3. **Credibility:** Leaders must uphold standards and be consistent.
4. **Accountability:** Individuals are professionally responsible for communicating concerns.
5. **Empowerment:** Individuals must feel as though they are being listened to and that their concerns will be taken seriously to effect change.
6. **Courage:** Individuals will question the risks to themselves and the consequences.
7. **Options:** The individual raising the concern must decide how and with whom he or she will raise the concern.

Activity

Reflect on Berry's (2004) framework and consider how you feel about the points raised in relation to your healthcare organisation. Consider the following questions:

- Do you feel that you understand the values within your healthcare organisation?
- Do the values of the healthcare organisation and your team conflict with your own?
- Do you feel able to identify breaches in these values?
- Do you feel engaged with your healthcare organisation?
- Are the leaders credible and are they consistent in their standards? Consider team leaders and more senior leaders within that healthcare organisation.
- Do you feel professionally responsible and accountable for raising concerns, and would you do so if the need arose?

GOV.UK (2013) provides information on UK government services and gives guidance on the protection employees have in relation to raising concerns. According to GOV.UK, you cannot be dismissed for raising concerns, but if you are you can claim unfair dismissal as long as the concerns qualify; 'qualifying disclosures' are discussed in the following material. The law protects employees, agency staff and those who are training within that organisation but who are not employed (including student nurses). However, those who are not employed can only claim for 'detrimental treatment' and not for unfair dismissal. If you do report a concern, you must be sure that there is truth in what you are reporting; otherwise, you will not be protected from dismissal under these rules. In addition, if you break the law by reporting concerns or if you breach legal or professional privileges, you will not be protected from dismissal.

The Public Interest Disclosure Act

The Public Interest Disclosure Act (PIDA) (1998) provides you with legal protection (1) to disclose information in the public interest and (2) if you bring action and are victimised as a result. The PIDA (1998) protects you if you are dismissed because you made a 'protected disclosure'; if so, it is likely you have been unfairly dismissed. Under this act, you have the right not to be subjected to any disadvantage by any act, or any failure to act, by your employer on the ground that you made a protected disclosure. Part IVA of the PIDA outlines which disclosures qualify for protection; a summary is provided in Box 11.4.

Box 11.4

Disclosures qualifying for protection (PIDA 1998, Part IVA)

To be 'protected', the employee must show at least one of the following in their disclosure:

a. That a criminal offence has been committed, is being committed or is likely to be committed,
b. That a person has failed, is failing or is likely to fail to comply with any legal obligation to which he is subject,
c. That a miscarriage of justice has occurred, is occurring or is likely to occur,
d. That the health or safety of any individual has been, is being or is likely to be endangered,
e. That the environment has been, is being or is likely to be damaged,
f. That information tending to show any matter falling within any one of the preceding paragraphs has been, is being or is likely to be deliberately concealed.

In all cases the disclosure must be made in good faith.

Confidentiality

It would be difficult to raise a concern without breaching confidentiality, and this seems to be an acceptable breach of this professional standard (Firtko and Jackson 2005). The PIDA (1998) will protect you for a breach of confidentiality outlined in any contract of employment if the disclosure is made in the interests of the public and satisfies the criteria of the disclosures qualifying for protection outlined in Box 11.4.

In terms of your confidentiality, although the law does not specifically require you to give your name when raising a concern, in the spirit of openness, it is generally recommended that you do give your name (CQC 2012; NMC 2013; RCN 2013). Your employer should allow for you to raise your concerns confidentially unless required by law and unless you give your consent for your name to be shared. You can raise a concern verbally, but the NMC (2013) stipulated that this should then be put into writing, and you should keep an accurate record of your concerns. If you wish for your name to be kept confidential, you must state this as soon as you raise your concern (CQC 2012; NMC 2013; RCN 2013). However, there might be practical or legal limitations to this anonymity.

Support from other organisations

As well as your university and your colleagues, there are other outside agencies you can contact for advice and support. PCAW is a whistle-blowing charity that can provide free and confidential advice to you if you are unsure whether to or how to raise a public concern. This advice relates to serious wrongdoings and risk of malpractice in the workplace. The PCAW website has further information (http://www.pcaw.org.uk/advice).

The RCN can also provide support to its members. For more details, visit the RCN website (http://www.rcn.org.uk/support/raising_concerns/a_guide_for_rcn_members).

The CQC is keen to hear from nurses who have serious concerns about standards of care. They provide guidance on how to contact them on their website (http://www.cqc.org.uk/sites/default/files/media/documents/20120117_whistleblowing_quick_guide_final_update.pdf).

Chapter summary

This chapter not only highlighted the difficulties in raising concerns and challenging poor practice but also emphasised the consequences of doing nothing. The concepts of integrity and courage to report concerns were also explored, as was the guidance available to support you in this task; seven points to consider in raising concerns were provided. You have a professional responsibility to protect people in your care by ensuring that they are safe and cared for to a high standard. There is a requirement under the NMC Code to report concerns you have about their care or any threats to these standards. This may require you to report a colleague, team or manager, which can be difficult. It is important that you remain focussed on those people who need you to advocate for them and protect them when they are at their most vulnerable.

References

Ahern, K., McDonald, S. 2002. The beliefs of nurses who were involved in a whistleblowing event. *Journal of Advanced Nursing* 38: 303–309.

Berry, B. 2004. Organizational culture: A framework and strategies for facilitating employee whistleblowing. *Employee Responsibilities and Rights Journal* 16(1): 1–11.

Care Quality Commission (CQC). 2012. *Whistleblowing: Guidance for Workers of Registered Care Providers*. Available from: http://www.cqc.org.uk/sites/default/files/media/documents/rp_poc_100494_20120410_v3_00_whistleblowing_guidance_for_employees_of_registered_providers_afte_pcaw_comments_with_changes_tracked_for_publication.pdf (accessed 17 October 2013).

Corley, M., Minick, P., Elswick, R.K., Jacobs, M. 2005. Nurse moral distress and ethical work environment. *Nursing Ethics* 12: 381–390.

Day L. 2007. Courage as a virtue necessary to good nursing practice. *American Journal of Critical Care* 16(6): 613–616.

Department of Health. 2013. *The NHS Constitution for England.* London: Department of Health. Available from: https://www.gov.uk/government/uploads/system/uploads/attachment_data/file/170656/NHS_Constitution.pdf (accessed 17 October 2013).

Edmonson, C. 2010. Moral courage and the nurse leader. *Online Journal of Issues in Nursing* 15(3). Available from: http://www.nursingworld.org/MainMenuCategories/ANAMarketplace/ANAPeriodicals/OJIN/TableofContents/Vol152010/No3-Sept-2010/Moral-Courage-for-Nurse-Leaders.html (accessed 17 October 2013).

Epstein, E.G., Hamric, A.B. 2009. Moral distress, moral residue and the crescendo effect. *Journal of Clinical Ethics* 20(4): 330–342.

Firtko, A., Jackson, D. 2005. Do the ends justify the means? Nursing and the dilemma of whistleblowing. *Australian Journal of Advanced Nursing* 23(1): 51–56.

Fry, S.T., Harvey, R.H., Hurley, A.C., Foley, B.J. 2002. Development of a model of moral distress in military nursing. *Nursing Ethics* 9: 373–387.

Gov.UK. 2013. Whistleblowing. Available from: https://www.gov.uk/whistleblowing/overview (accessed 20 April 2014)

Griffith, R., Tengnah, C. 2012. Further legal protection needed for nurses who report poor practice. *British Journal of Community Nursing* 17: 287–290.

Hanna, D.R. 2004. Moral distress: The state of the science. *Research and Theory for Nursing Practice* 18: 73–93.

Jackson, D., Peters, K., Hutchinson, M., Edenborough, M., Luck, L., Wilkes, L. 2011. Exploring confidentiality in the context of nurse whistle blowing: Issues for nurse managers. *Journal of Nursing Management* 19: 655–663.

Jameton, A. 1984. *Nursing Practice: The Ethical Issues.* Englewood Cliffs, NJ: Prentice Hall.

Kelly, B. 1996. Hospital nursing: 'It's a battle!' A follow-up study of English graduate nurses. *Journal of Advanced Nursing* 24(5): 1063–1069.

Kelly, B. 1998. Preserving moral integrity: A follow-up study with new graduate nurses (experience before and throughout the nursing career). *Journal of Advanced Nursing* 28(5): 1134–1145.

Laabs, C. 2011. Perceptions of moral integrity: Contradictions in need of explanation. *Nursing Ethics* 18(3): 431–440.

Lachman, V.D. 2007. Moral courage: A virtue in need of development? *MedSurg Nursing* 16(2): 131–133.

LaSala, C.A., Bjarnason, D. 2010. Creating workplace environments that support moral courage. *Online Journal of Issues in Nursing* 15:3. Available from: http://www.nursingworld.org/MainMenuCategories/ANAMarketplace/ANAPeriodicals/OJIN/TableofContents/Vol152010/No3-Sept-2010/Workplace-Environments-and-Moral-Courage.html (accessed 17 October 2013).

Lindh, I.B., da Silva, A.B., Berg, A., Severinsson, E. 2010. Courage and nursing practice: A theoretical analysis. *Nursing Ethics* 17: 551–565.

Lindh, I.B., Severinsson, I.E., Berg, A. 2009. Nurses' moral strength: A hermeneutic inquiry in nursing practice. *Journal of Advanced Nursing* 65: 1882–1890.

Moore, L., McAuliffe, E. 2010. Is inadequate response to whistleblowing perpetuating a culture of silence in hospitals? *Clinical Governance* 15: 166–178.

Near, J.P., Miceli, M.P. 1985. Organizational dissidence: The case of whistle-blowing. *Journal of Business Ethics* 4(1): 1–16.

Nursing and Midwifery Council (NMC). 2008. *The Code: Standards of Conduct, Performance and Ethics for Nurses and Midwives.* London: NMC.

Nursing and Midwifery Council (NMC). 2009. *Guidance on Professional Conduct for Nursing and Midwifery Students.* London: NMC.

Nursing and Midwifery Council (NMC). 2013. *Raising Concerns Guidance for Nurses and Midwives.* London: NMC.

Public Interest Disclosure Act (PIDA). 1998. Available from: http://www.legislation.gov.uk/ukpga/1998/23/introduction (accessed 17 October 2013).

Royal College of Nursing (RCN). 2011. *Nurses Still Afraid to Blow the Whistle.* Available from: http://www.rcn.org.uk/newsevents/press_releases/uk/nurses_still_afraid_to_blow_the_whistle_-_rcn (accessed 17 October 2013).

Royal College of Nursing (RCN). 2013. *Raising Concerns: A Guide for RCN Members*. Available from: http://www.rcn.org.uk/__data/assets/pdf_file/0015/510180/004391.pdf (accessed 17 October 2013).

Webster, G., Baylis, F. 2000. Moral residue. In Rubin, S.B., and Zoloth, L. (eds.), *Margin of Error: The Ethics of Mistakes in the Practice of Medicine.* Hagerstown, MD: University Publishing Group, 217–232.

Wilmot, S. 2000. Nurses and whistle-blowing: The ethical issues. *Journal of Advanced Nursing* 32(5): 1051–1057.

12

Promoting best practice and continuing professional development

Introduction

This chapter focusses on the professional requirement to engage in continuing professional development and lifelong learning in order to deliver and promote care that is based on the best available evidence. Recent reports have highlighted the accountability of nurses and other healthcare professionals for the quality of care provided to patients (Francis 2013), so it is essential that nurses continue to develop their practice and apply best evidence in care delivery, underpinned by their professional values. The nature of best evidence is discussed as well as how to access and apply best evidence in practice. The chapter explores ways of developing and improving your own practice as a professional nurse, from the point of registration onwards. A culture in which curiosity is encouraged for nurses is important (Eason 2010), and as a registered nurse you will be able to contribute to developing a culture of learning and professional development.

Learning outcomes

By the end of this chapter, you will be able to

- Discuss the professional requirement to engage in lifelong learning and deliver and promote care that is based on the best available evidence;
- Recognise the need to access, appraise and implement best evidence for practice;
- Appreciate and engage with opportunities to develop as a professional nurse to continually improve your own practice.

Maintaining and developing professional knowledge

The Nursing and Midwifery Council (NMC) (2008) requires that nurses must deliver care that is based on the best available evidence or best practice. The NMC (2008) also expects nurses to keep their knowledge and skills up to date throughout their working lives, participating in appropriate learning activities to develop competence and performance. The NMC (2011) guidance for post-registration education and practice (Prep) aims to help registrants provide a high standard of practice and care, keep up to date with new developments in practice, and think and reflect and demonstrate that they are keeping up to date and developing their practice. As discussed in Chapter 2, the NMC will publish an enhanced Code towards the end of 2014, but the requirement to deliver evidence-based practice (EBP) and to engage in continuing professional development will remain a key theme. Chapter 2 explains the NMC's Prep requirements in more detail and the NMC's proposals for revalidation of nurses and midwives, scheduled to commence in 2015.

Activity

Consider: What could happen if a registered nurse does not engage in continuing professional development?

The evidence base for practice is constantly developing, and registered nurses must base their practice on current, up-to-date evidence to ensure that people receive the best possible care. There is a public expectation that individual nurses and midwives are up to date and fit to practise at all times (NMC 2013), so a failure to be so will diminish public confidence in these professions. A desire to incorporate the newest evidence into nursing practice is a component of lifelong learning (Eason 2010). Courey et al. (2006) argued that the evolution of nursing as a profession requires the development of evidence-based practice linked to outcomes; therefore, nurses must be able to access and evaluate professional literature. The context for nursing practice is also continually changing; for example, legislation, health policy and professional guidance affect the way that nurses practise and deliver care. Chapter 10 illustrates this point well, as policy and legislation relevant to the safeguarding of children and adults is continually developed and revised, often as a result of public inquiries.

The overall aim of a lifelong learning approach is to ensure that clinical practice is evidence based, skilled, and led appropriately (Petaloti 2009). As a registered nurse, your lifelong learning will be supported through continuous professional development (CPD) activities. Gopee's (2005) literature review highlighted key reasons that lifelong learning is an important aspect of professional practice:

- the need for practitioners to be self-directed so that they can access the required knowledge for their practice as and when it is needed;
- the mandatory requirement for continuing professional education;
- the evolving nature of health care and practice (for example, relating to technological advancements) with the associated need for professional development;
- the relationship between professional development and the shift along the continuum of novice to expert for the enhancement of clinical practice.

In addition, Eason (2010) asserted that lifelong learning supports critical thinking, can enhance nurses' satisfaction with their professional role and supports the desire to apply the newest evidence into nursing practice. She further asserted that a culture in which educational growth is supported and promoted is vital for advancing nursing as a profession. How nurses and midwives interact with the concept of lifelong learning is varied, and requirements from the NMC are flexible.

Activity

List all the ways through which you could continue your learning and keep yourself up to date as a registered nurse.

When next in practice, ask some registered nurses questions related to the following:

- How they continue their learning and keep themselves up to date
- Tips they can give you for keeping up to date and carrying on your learning after registration

A few ways you might have thought of include

- Work-based learning (e.g. reflective practice, reviewing clinical audit results and incident reports, feedback from patients/families).
- Reading professional bulletins (e.g. from the Royal College of Nursing [RCN] and the NMC).
- Attending seminars, journal clubs, training, post-registration courses, lectures or conferences. These may be organised internally in your organisation, in partner universities or in other forums; look for posters, set up alerts or join e-mail circulation lists for organisations that interest you.

- Maintaining a continually inquiring mind and thirst for knowing more. When you encounter anything in practice that you are unsure of, access available resources (e.g. colleagues, your organisation's intranet, the National Institute for Health and Clinical Excellence [NICE] website, the RCN website, journal articles [using an electronic database], specialist websites).
- Talking to experts. These experts could be colleagues (e.g. nurses in your own team, specialist nurses, multi-disciplinary team members) or experts by experience (service users or carers).
- Taking on a link nurse role. You may have the chance to be a link nurse or champion (e.g. for infection control, tissue viability, dementia, dignity). This will give you the chance to talk regularly with experts (e.g. lead nurse for dementia) and to meet with other staff across the organisation who are interested in this topic.

Reflective practice

Developing your reflective skills will help you to learn and develop your practice so that you optimise your learning. Dewey, an educational theorist, argued that we do not 'learn by doing' but by 'doing and realizing what came of what we did' (Dewey 1929, p. 367). Dewey's theories were developed further by Kolb and Fry (1975) and then more fully by Kolb (1984). The theory of how we learn from experience is often referred to as 'experiential learning' and is portrayed as a cycle (Kolb 1984). The process starts at the point of a concrete experience or event, after which observations and reflections occur, followed by abstract conceptualisation, where new ideas are developed, linked to other knowledge and experience, and then the new knowledge arising from the experience is tested in a new situation. This new experience then starts the experiential learning cycle once again.

Reflection enables you to consider what you did and why and provides opportunities to develop knowledge from experience and link theory and practice. Knowledge gained from reflection on practice has been termed 'practical knowledge' (Schön 1987), and reflection can enable the uncovering of knowledge embedded in practice (Lawler 1991). Reflecting on your practice helps you to examine your experience and consider other explanations for what happened and alternative ways of doing things (Howartson-Jones 2010). Reflection may occur during the experience ('reflection-in-action') or following the experience ('reflection-on-action') (Schön 1991). Reflection is particularly relevant to professional growth in a practice-based discipline such as nursing, as nursing knowledge is embedded in experience, and learning through experience is essential to the practice of professional nursing (Brunero and Stein-Parbury 2008).

There are various models of reflective practice that have been developed to give structure and focus. For example, the Gibbs (1988) reflective cycle includes the components shown in Figure 12.1, which you work through in a cyclical manner to reflect on a particular experience.

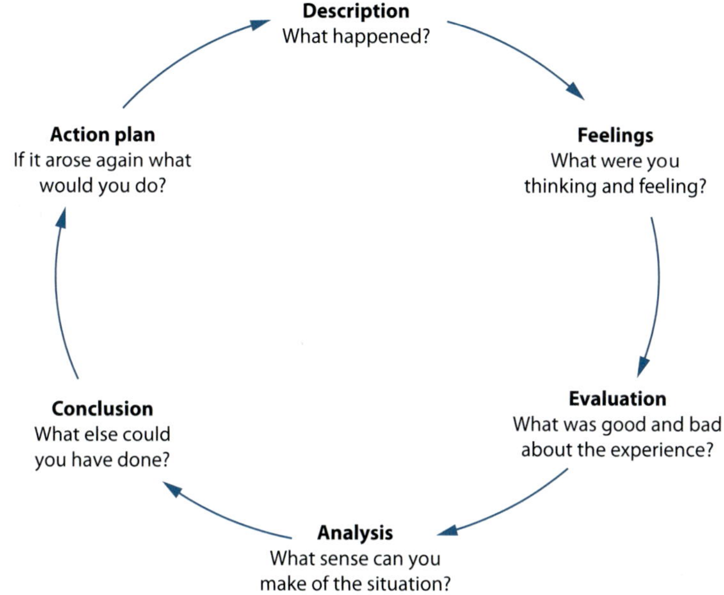

Figure 12.1 Gibbs reflective cycle.

Other reflective models include those of Palmer et al. (1994), who suggested a series of cue questions, and Borton's (1970) developmental framework, which comprises three areas of focus:

- **What?** (description of what happened);
- **So what?** (the context–theory and knowledge building);
- **Now what?** (action–what to do next).

Driscoll (2007) developed Borton's (1970) model in a nursing context and linked it to an experiential learning cycle. Johns (2013) has developed a model for structured reflection that has been refined over many years. The model aims to assist practitioners to 'access the depth and breadth of reflection to facilitate learning through experience' (p. 37); see Johns (2013) for his current version and underpinning theories. Wigens and Heathershaw (2013) considered that it is important not to use reflective models as checklists and to avoid ritualization in their use.

There are many texts focussed on reflective practice available, so do access these for further reading on this topic.

Best evidence for practice

Nurses must deliver and promote care that is based on the best available evidence. It is therefore essential to be able to identify gaps in knowledge about evidence and know how to address these on an ongoing basis, as evidence is continually updating.

Read Box 12.1 and consider the questions posed.

Box 12.1

Practice scenario: identifying and addressing knowledge gaps

Carl is a third-year mental health student who is in his first week of a placement in a community mental health team. With his mentor, he visits a woman, Mary, who has a long history of depression and has been referred for a re-assessment. She also has a long-standing pituitary disorder. Mary expresses concern that the medication she is taking for her depression and her pituitary condition have side effects and are doing her 'more harm than good'. During the assessment, Carl records Mary's blood pressure, which is 150/90 mm Hg; she has no history of hypertension. Carl's mentor suggests that Mary needs to make an appointment with the practice nurse to have further blood pressure monitoring as her blood pressure is 'higher than it should be'.

After the visit, Carl's mentor asks him questions about Mary concerning the medication she is taking and the side effects, how a pituitary condition might affect mental health, and the normal blood pressure range. Carl finds that he is struggling to answer some of these questions. His mentor advises him that an important part of being a safe professional is to acknowledge gaps in his knowledge so that he can address these. He suggests Carl write an action plan for what he needs to learn and how he will go about this.

Questions

1. Why is it important for safety that a nurse acknowledges gaps in knowledge or skills?
2. If a service user asks a question that you cannot answer, what would you say as a student and as a registered nurse?
3. What resources could Carl access to address the gaps in his knowledge?
4. What might constitute best evidence?

Although the scenario in Box 12.1 is based on a third-year student, remember that you could encounter such situations as a registered nurse. There are many resources available to healthcare professionals to develop and update their knowledge. Here are examples of resources that Carl could access for information:

- The British Hypertension Society website (http://www.bhsoc.org/)
- The Pituitary Foundation website (http://www.pituitary.org.uk/)

- The British National Formulary website (http://www.bnf.org)
- Expert practitioners (e.g. pharmacists have expert knowledge about side effects of medication and drug interactions)
- Textbooks: to look up information on pharmacology, pituitary disorders, depression
- The National Institute for Health and Clinical Excellence (NICE) evidence-based guidelines and quality standards (see http://www.nice.org.uk)
- The Cochrane Library: online resource that provides systematic reviews of research on different topics

NICE and the Cochrane Library systematic reviews are regularly updated, so always access the most up-to-date versions. An excellent source of information is the Evidence Search Health and Social Care website (http://www.evidence.nhs.uk), which includes access to resources for evidence-based practice and a facility to search for evidence. Often, National Health Service (NHS) trusts and other healthcare organisations have their own clinical guidelines, based on best evidence, to assist nurses and other healthcare professionals to implement evidence-based practice in the local context.

Activity

- Find out about how evidence-based clinical guidelines and policies are developed in your organisation. Is there a committee? Who are the members?
- Where are the policies and guidelines kept?
- Access one of these documents (ask your mentor's assistance) and examine it for its evidence base and currency (date published and review date).

No one can know everything, and the knowledge base for nursing practice and health care is continually developing and expanding. Therefore, it is essential to be able to know how to find information and to have the motivation and commitment to address your knowledge and skills deficits. Not being aware of or acknowledging the gaps in your knowledge and skills could endanger patients as you will not be able to provide them with safe and best-quality care. Your professional values that underpin your practice should guide you in such situations: Honesty and a real commitment to do what is best for people in your care must take priority over any personal feelings of disappointment or embarrassment associated with admitting that you do not know something. So, as a student and as a registered nurse, it is really important to

- acknowledge the limitations of your knowledge and skill;
- have the skills, motivation and commitment to rectify deficits in your knowledge and skills;

- seek expert guidance to ensure that your patients have the best possible care.

If a service user asks you a question that you cannot answer, it is better to be honest about the limits of your knowledge, but importantly you then need to explain how you will help the patient, for example, by consulting with an expert or accessing a reliable information source.

Care should be based on best available evidence, which may be derived from research, but it may also be based on experience and through reflection on practice (as discussed previously). Benner (1984) identified that practice is always more complex and presents many more realities than theory ever can, and she highlighted the value of theory derived from practice. Nurses are accountable for their actions, so they must be able to explain the knowledge base underpinning their practice. Benner (1984) explored how expert nurses develop knowledge from their practice, learning to recognise, for example, subtle changes in people's conditions.

Evidence-based practice

This next activity prompts you to reflect on the evidence underpinning your nursing practice.

Activity

Reflect on one intervention that you have recently used in nursing practice. Consider:

- What evidence informed this intervention?
- Where did this evidence come from?
- How did you judge the quality of the evidence that you used in practice?

Cullum et al. (2008) defined evidence-based nursing as 'the application of valid, relevant, research-based information in nurse decision-making' (p. 2). Barker (2013) reviewed various definitions and identified four types of evidence for nursing practice: research, clinical experience, service user/carer perspectives and the local context of care.

The evidence-based practice literature refers to a hierarchy of evidence:

1. High quality meta-analyses/systematic reviews of randomized controlled trials (RCTs);
2. Well-designed RCTs;
3. Other types of experimental studies (e.g. pre-test, post-test);

4. Non-experimental studies;
5. Descriptive studies, expert reports.

NICE guidelines, and other clinical guidelines, use meta-analyses/systematic reviews whenever possible as the basis for their evidence-based guidelines. An RCT uses an experimental approach to determine the effectiveness of an intervention (e.g. a medicine, a wound dressing, a method of giving patient information). Key features of an RCT are randomization and control. Therefore, the people taking part in the RCT are randomly allocated to either the group of individuals who receive the intervention (the independent variable) or to a control group of people who do not receive the intervention (e.g. in the case of a medicine trial, they would be given a placebo). The results of the trial derive from measuring the effect of the independent variable on one or more dependent variables, for example, the expected effect of the drug in the case of a drug trial or wound-healing measures in a trial of a wound dressing. The trial is set up to control as much as possibly any factors that might confound the results, so the sample will meet specific criteria and thus reduce the effect of additional factors that might affect the effect of the independent variable. In the case of wound dressing trials, people with diabetes are often excluded from taking part as their diabetes is an additional factor ('extraneous variable') that could affect their wound healing. Unfortunately, this has led to many types of wound dressing not having been tested adequately on people with diabetes. Exclusion of individuals to achieve control has led to certain groups of people being excluded from opportunities to participate in research, which has ethical implications. Nevertheless, the RCT is considered a particularly reliable form of evidence, and a systematic review uses a prescribed method to identify and critically appraise RCTs on a particular topic.

The Cochrane Library (http://www.thecochranelibrary.com) aims to provide high-quality, independent evidence to inform healthcare decision-making. The library contains databases of systematic reviews on an increasing number of topics.

While traditionally the Cochrane Library's systematic reviews appraised only RCTs, recently Gülmezoglu et al. (2013) reported on an 'important milestone' for the Cochrane Library, which published, for the first time, a review of qualitative studies. The topic was a review of the barriers and facilitators to the implementation of lay health worker programmes. Gülmezoglu et al. (2013) argued that the synthesis of qualitative evidence makes an important contribution to the knowledge available to organisations such as the World Health Organisation that are developing international recommendations on public health topics. In particular, qualitative evidence may give insights into patient experience and likely acceptability of a particular intervention.

Activity

Go to the Cochrane Library website (http://www.thecochranelibrary.com) and search for systematic reviews on topics relevant to the scenario in Box 12.1:

1. Hypertension management
2. Pituitary disorder
3. Depression

Access one review on each topic and read the abstract, taking note of how many studies were selected for review and the final conclusion of this evidence.

In nursing practice, the notion that systematic reviews and RCTs should always be at the top of the hierarchy of evidence has attracted some criticism, as nursing practice requires multiple ways of knowing (Barker 2013). There are many nursing topics for which there is no conclusive evidence based on systematic reviews of RCTs. Furthermore, the application of the results of a systematic review must take into account the individual and the context of care. For example, a particular pressure-relieving mattress might have been shown to be effective in preventing pressure ulcers and be recommended in evidence-based guidelines, but the use of the mattress in practice must take into account patient preference and effect on their comfort and overall care (e.g. mobilisation goals). Barker (2013) also reported that critics of evidence-based practice argue that generalised evidence-based guidelines detract from a person-centred approach (see Chapter 7), hence that is why it is important to review evidence in the light of the individual and the individual's situation. A collaborative group that supports evidence-based practice and has a stronger nursing focus is the Joanna Briggs Institute (JBI), which was established in Australia. The JBI takes a broader approach to consideration of evidence to underpin practice.

Barker (2013) presented various models for applying evidence-based practice and she identified the following skills and components:

- The ability to identify what counts as appropriate evidence is required.
- Formulation of the search topic into an answerable question to focus the evidence gathering is the key to a good literature search; using the PICO format (population, intervention, comparison, outcome) can help to focus the evidence search (see Norris 2010).
- Development of a strategy for searching for evidence and familiarisation with search engines and databases that will assist with the search for evidence, for example, CINAHL (Cumulative Index to Nursing and Allied Health Literature), MEDLINE, PschINFO, BNI (British Nurse

Index) and SCOPUS are commonly used when searching for evidence for nursing practice.

- Critical appraisal of the evidence is an essential step in order to make a judgement regarding the quality of the evidence. There are many useful appraisal guidelines available; see the UK Critical Appraisal Skills Programme (CASP) (http://www.casp-uk.net), which includes checklists for appraising different types of research.
- Clinical expertise will help to contexualise the evidence.
- Consideration of patient preferences: see Chapter 7 ('Person-Centred and Holistic Nursing Care') and Chapter 8 ('Working in Partnership with Service Users, Carers, and Families, particularly the section on shared decision-making).
- Application of the evidence to the context of care delivery.
- Implementation of the evidence in practice.

Many articles have debated the difficulties associated with implementation of evidence in practice; the embedding of changes in staff behaviour are always challenging. What appear to be small changes in practice can involve many different disciplines and changes to whole systems. Service improvement methodology has been used successfully to map current processes and try out and refine changes on a small scale using repeated Plan-Do-Study-Act cycles (Langley et al. 2009).

One method of applying EBP is the use of care bundles. A care bundle is a set of evidence-based interventions that, used together, improve patient outcomes. As an example, the NHS Institute for Innovation and Improvement (2009) identified four key elements for a care bundle to prevent pressure ulcers, which used the acronym SKIN: **s**urface, **k**eep moving, **in**continence and **n**utrition. Other examples of care bundles used in practice relate to pre-operative care, prevention of falls, dementia care, ventilator care, discharge of patients and catheter care.

Activity

When next in practice, investigate what, if any, care bundles are being used. Find out what their elements are and what their evidence base is. Through observing in practice and asking your mentor, respond to the following questions:

- How well has the care bundle been embedded into everyday practice?
- What have been the facilitators to implementing the care bundle?
- What have been the barriers to implementing the care bundle?

Developing as a professional nurse

Nurses, midwives and other health professionals are, from the point of registration, autonomous and accountable (Department of Health [DH] 2010), but there has been increasing recognition of the benefits of supporting newly registered staff and assisting them in consolidating their learning. Harrison-White and Simons (2013) reported on the experiences of newly qualified children's nurses who found that the role change had been fraught, particularly the increased responsibilities and dealing with the expectations of more experienced staff. The 'reality shock' for newly qualified nurses is well documented (Duchscher 2009), and support in the first year can assist the transition.

Read Nabila's scenario in Box 12.2 and consider the questions posed. Preceptorship, clinical supervision and appraisal are explored in the next sections; as you read this material, consider how these might support Nabila as a registered nurse and think about yourself and your future development following registration.

Box 12.2

Practice scenario: professional development and support

Nabila is a newly qualified children's nurse, and she has just started in a post on a children's ward. She is excited about her job but is also feeling anxious. She will be starting on the trust's inter-professional preceptorship course in a month's time, and she is looking forward to the course. The ward sister tells Nabila that they are going to be introducing clinical supervision on the ward in the near future. Nabila also learns that all staff on the ward have an annual appraisal at which their performance and development are reviewed.

Questions

1. What is preceptorship, and how might this benefit Nabila?
2. What is 'clinical supervision'? How might clinical supervision support staff development and safe professional practice?
3. What is the purpose of appraisal? How does appraisal link to professional development?

Preceptorship

Staff working in the NHS are entitled to 12 months of preceptorship following registration (NHS Staff Council 2013). In 2010, the DH published the *Preceptorship Framework for Newly Registered Nurses, Midwives and Allied Health Professionals*, in which preceptorship is defined as

> *a period of structured transition for the newly registered practitioner during which time he or she will be supported by a preceptor, to develop their confidence as an autonomous professional, refine skills, values and behaviours to continue on their journey of lifelong learning.*
>
> (p. 11)

A preceptor is defined in the framework as

> *a registered practitioner who has been given a formal responsibility to support a newly registered practitioner through preceptorship.*
>
> (DH 2010, p. 6)

Be aware that in the international literature, the term *preceptor* is sometimes used more broadly to include registered nurses who support nursing students, referred to as 'mentors' in the United Kingdom. The DH's (2010) framework emphasises the need for all newly registered practitioners to experience a structured and supportive preceptorship period, acknowledging that the immediate period following registration can be a challenging time and that good support and guidance are essential. The overall aim is for the registered practitioner to become

> *an effective, confident and fully autonomous registered individual, who is able to deliver high quality care for patients, clients and service users.*
>
> (DH 2010, p. 21)

The DH (2010) identified that preceptorship can reap benefits for both individuals and organisations because if the transition to being a registered professional is managed successfully, staff will provide effective care more quickly and retention within the professions will be increased, leading to a greater contribution to patient care. Preceptorship supports well the concept of lifelong learning, as it sets the scene for the continuing of learning and development following registration. Following a review with stakeholders, the DH (2010) identified elements of preceptorship for newly qualified practitioners (see Box 12.3) and outlined the attributes for an effective preceptor, highlighting that these are likely to take up to 2 years to develop post-registration. Ford et al. (2013) found that preceptors recognised their professional responsibility to those entering the profession and were committed to the development of these learners. The preceptor will know the organisation and can offer invaluable support during adjustment to being a registered professional. Wigens and Heathershaw (2013) identified that newly qualified nurses need to review their achievements to date; understand expectations of them; adapt to their new role and develop new skills; continue to learn and develop their practice; effectively deliver patient care and feel valued as part of the team.

There are a number of examples of preceptorship programmes that have been reported in journal articles, and some of these include evaluation.

Box 12.3

Elements of preceptorship for newly qualified practitioners

- Opportunity to apply and develop the knowledge, skills and values already learned.
- Develop specific competences that relate to the preceptee's role.
- Access support in embedding the values and expectations of the profession.
- Personalised programme of development that includes post-registration learning, e.g. leadership, management and effectively working within a multi-disciplinary team.
- Opportunity to reflect on practice and receive constructive feedback.
- Take responsibility for individual learning and development by learning how to 'manage self'.
- Continuation of life-long learning.
- Enables the embracement of the principles of the NHS Constitution.

From Department of Health (DH). 2013. *Preceptorship Framework for Newly Registered Nurses, Midwives and Allied Health Professionals. Nursing.* Gateway reference 13889. p. 13. Available from: http://webarchive.nationalarchives.gov.uk/20130107105354/http://www.dh.gov.uk/prod_consum_dh/groups/dh_digitalassets/@dh/@en/@abous/documents/digitalasset/dh_114116.pdf (accessed 16 October 2013).

For example, Leigh et al.'s (2005) preceptorship programme for newly qualified nurses apparently led to increased recruitment and retention of newly qualified nurses, who self-reported increased levels of confidence. Daylan (2012) provided a first-hand account of the daunting experience of being a newly qualified nurse but how her trust's preceptorship programme supported her as she gained confidence in her new role. Harrison-White and Simons (2013) also argued that the transition from student to staff nurse can be achieved more smoothly with the support of a preceptorship programme.

A range of methods exists through which preceptorship programmes could be delivered, but core elements should be theoretical learning and supervision/guided reflection (DH 2010). Many NHS trusts organise preceptorship from a multi-professional perspective as it is beneficial for staff who work interprofessionally to also learn together, as discussed in Chapter 9. Typically, as well as allocating a preceptor to each newly qualified practitioner, a preceptorship programme will comprise some set study days, which offer peer support, and there may be workbooks or other distance learning materials, with competencies to be achieved. As an example, Chapman (2013) reported on a flexible 'roll-on, roll-off' preceptorship pathway for all new nursing and allied health professional registrants. Staff stay on the pathway for 6–12 months, depending on their personal development needs, achievement of competencies and appraisal outcomes. In another published example, Morgan et al. (2012) reported on a structured preceptorship programme that is linked to the core dimensions in the Knowledge and Skills Framework (KSF; see the section on appraisal) and includes the allocation of a preceptor, classroom-based learning, group work, self-directed learning, portfolio development and regular review meetings. Some preceptorship programmes will expect preceptees to carry out a project, for example, a service improvement project, possibly in a group.

Activity

Talk to a nurse who qualified in the past year and ask them:

- What were their experiences of preceptorship, and how did preceptorship help their transition?
- Do they have any tips for you to help ease your transition from student to registered nurse status?

Clinical supervision

Clinical supervision is mandatory in many professions (e.g. midwifery, counselling), but within the nursing profession, its implementation has been varied. Brunero and Stein-Parbury (2008) found evidence that clinical supervision has been established in some areas of nursing practice for some time (e.g. mental health nursing, end-of-life care), but that it is gradually being applied to other clinical contexts. There has often been misinterpretation of what clinical supervision means, with the assumption that it is about monitoring or overseeing performance rather than development of individuals. The Care Quality Commission (CQC) (2013) acknowledged that different terms may be used (e.g. 'professional supervision', 'peer supervision', 'developmental supervision', 'reflective supervision' or just 'supervision) but emphasised that the process is separate from managerial supervision through performance monitoring and appraisal (see next section).

Proctor (1986) (cited by Brunero and Stein-Parbury 2008) identified three functions of clinical supervision:

- **Formative**: an educative activity aimed at increasing knowledge, self-awareness, creativity and innovation;
- **Normative:** enables the development of consistency in approaches to patient care (i.e. 'norms' or standards of practice) and assists the development of strategies to manage the professional accountability and quality issues in nursing;

- **Restorative**: promotes validation and support for colleagues through peer feedback and manages the emotional response to patient care.

Using Proctor's (1986) framework in their analysis, Brunero and Stein-Parbury (2008) identified that clinical supervision provided peer support and stress relief for nurses (restorative function), promoted professional accountability (normative function) and supported skills and knowledge development (formative function). Brunero and Stein-Parbury (2008) identified that reflection is the primary cognitive process during clinical supervision as nurses can think back on clinical experiences so that they can deepen their understanding or identify areas for further improvement.

As regards the evidence base for clinical supervision, from a review of the literature, Brunero and Stein-Parbury (2008) asserted that there is sufficient evidence for clinical supervision to be implemented in nursing. However, Buus and Gonge's (2009) systematic review of clinical supervision in mental health nursing concluded there was insufficient evidence as studies were often too small scale and there were varied models in place. Bégat and Severinsson's (2006) synthesis of three studies of clinical supervision led to the conclusion that clinical supervision had a positive influence on nurses' experiences of well-being and that nurses attending clinical supervision reported increased satisfaction with their psychosocial work environment. In a study of nurses working in a dementia unit, clinical supervision was found to address support in professional and personal growth, ethical issues, clinical practice and education (Berg and Welander Hansson 2000).

Bishop (2007) identified that the key aspect of clinical supervision that is not present in other support systems is the element of peer review and supportive challenge. She argued that clinical supervision can bring out the 'sharpness in clinical practice–that extra awareness which derives from shared learning with colleagues' (p. 3). Bishop (2007) also highlighted that clinical supervision can offer a framework to support nurses with their professional accountability, although it is important to emphasise that nurses remain accountable for their own practice.

There has been increasing acknowledgement that the well-being of healthcare professionals has a positive impact on the quality of care delivered. Accordingly, ways of supporting staff, including clinical supervision, are attracting more attention. The CQC (2013) explained that clinical supervision provides an opportunity for professionals to

- Reflect on and review their practice;
- Discuss individual cases in depth;
- Change or modify their practice and identify training and continuing development needs.

The CQC (2013) set out the purpose of clinical supervision as provision of a safe and confidential environment for staff to reflect on and discuss their practice and their personal and professional responses to their work, thus supporting staff in their development. The potential benefits of clinical supervision are summarised in Table 12.1. The CQC (2013) asserted that clinical supervision might particularly benefit staff who work with people

Table 12.1 Benefits of Clinical Supervision

	Benefits
Staff	• Can help staff to manage the work-related personal and professional demands through providing an environment in which they can explore their own personal and emotional reactions to their work. • Can allow staff to reflect on and challenge their own practice in a safe and confidential environment and receive feedback on their skills (separately from managerial considerations). • Can form part of staff professional development and help to identify developmental needs. • Can contribute towards meeting professional body requirements for continuing professional development.
Service users	• Helps to ensure that people who use services and their carers receive high-quality care at all times from staff who can manage the personal and emotional impact of their practice.
Providers	• Can support the culture of the organisation, which sets the tone, values and behaviours expected of individuals. • Along with good practices in recruitment, induction and training, helps ensure that staff have the right skills, attitudes and support to provide high-quality services. • Associated with higher levels of job satisfaction, improved retention, reduced turnover and staff effectiveness. • May increase employees' perceptions of organisational support and improve their commitment to an organisation's vision and goals. • A way for providers to fulfil their duty of care to staff. • Linked to good clinical governance by helping to support quality improvement, managing risks, and increasing accountability. • Supports CPD, which is a requirement for registration in many professions and therefore ensures the workforce remains registered.

Source: Summarised from Care Quality Commission (CQC). 2013. *Supporting Information and Guidance: Supporting Effective Clinical Supervision*. pp. 5–6. Available from: http://www.cqc.org.uk/sites/default/files/media/documents/20130625_800734_v1_00_supporting_information-effective_clinical_supervision_for_publication.pdf (accessed 24 November 2013).

with complex and challenging needs, for example, people with a learning disability and challenging behaviour or mental health needs, supporting them in maintaining good relationships with service users and carers.

Supervision may be carried out on a one-to-one basis or in a group and should be carried out on a regular basis (CQC 2013). Supervisors should have the skills, qualifications, experience and knowledge of the area of practice required to undertake their role effectively (CQC 2013). Effective supervision relies on trust; therefore, normally the content of the session should be confidential, but if concerns arise in the course of supervision about a staff member's conduct, competence or physical or mental health, the supervisor may need to disclose information from a supervision session to an appropriate person, such as the staff member's line manager (CQC 2013).

Brunero and Stein-Parbury (2008) emphasised the peer-educative function of clinical supervision and that, through their participation, nurses can provide feedback and input to their colleagues to assist them to increase their understanding about clinical issues. They further explained that clinical supervision provides nurses with an opportunity to improve patient care in particular for specific individuals but also in relation to maintaining overall standards of care. Clinical supervision also provides an opportunity for nurses to demonstrate active support for each other as professional colleagues and that through sharing experiences they realise that they are 'not alone' in their feelings and perceptions of practice, thus providing them with reassurance and validation (Brunero and Stein-Parbury 2008).

Appraisal

The NHS Constitution (DH 2013, p. 13) sets out that employees can expect to be provided with 'personal development, access to appropriate education and training for their jobs, and line management support to enable them to fulfil their potential'. One structure that supports staff development is an annual appraisal with their line manager, which provides an important opportunity to review both current performance and professional development. All NHS employees are entitled to an annual appraisal (see NHS Employers' website at http://www.nhsemployers.org). If you are employed outside the NHS (e.g. social care, voluntary or private sector), you should check what the organisation will offer you to support your development. Good employment practices would be that you have opportunities for professional development and have at least an annual review.

To obtain the most from appraisal, you need to invest some time and ensure that you prepare adequately. The NHS Employers' website provides information for appraisees as well as appraisers, including tips about preparation through reflecting on your performance, development and achievement over the past year. You and your manager will, following the review of your work, set SMART (specific, measurable, achievable, relevant, timebound) objectives for you to work towards.

The Knowledge and Skills Framework (KSF) was established when the NHS Agenda for Change Bands 1–9 pay scale was implemented in 2004 (RCN 2005). The KSF set out core dimensions for every job in the NHS:

1. Communication
2. Personal and people development
3. Health, safety and security
4. Service improvement
5. Quality
6. Equality and diversity

There are further specific dimensions that relate to parts of particular posts. The KSF remains part of the Agenda for Change national terms and conditions and is a development tool for healthcare workers that contributes to decisions about pay progression and provides a structure to help staff develop their careers. Your appraisal is likely to focus on your performance in the KSF in relation to your job role. Individual NHS trusts will also incorporate other factors; for example, the trust's values (discussed in Chapter 1) might be incorporated into your appraisal. Good practice is that you should have an interim/midyear review with ongoing discussion about your progress against the objectives, your performance and your development.

Chapter summary

Important values for professional nursing practice include a commitment to lifelong learning and to ensuring that practice is up to date and based on the best available evidence. As a registered nurse, you must be aware of your limitations and any gaps in your knowledge and skills so that you can take steps to address these through accessing, appraising and applying best evidence in your practice. The transition from student status to confident registered nurse can be daunting. You need to ensure that you engage with the support processes that are available, such as preceptorship, and use the appraisal process as a structure to plan your development. You should appreciate and reflect on ways of developing as a professional nurse so that you continually improve your own practice. Above all, ensure that you make a real commitment to continual learning; listen to and learn from patients, carers and colleagues and use the many resources available to keep yourself up to date.

References

Barker, J. 2013. *Evidence-Based Practice for Nurses*. 2nd ed. London: Sage.

Bégat, I., Severinsson, E. 2006. Reflection on how clinical nursing supervision enhances nurses' experiences of well-being related to their psychosocial work environment. *Journal of Nursing Management* 14: 610–616.

Benner, P. 1984. *From Novice to Expert.* Boston: Addison-Wesley.

Berg, A., Welander Hansson, U. 2000. Dementia care nurses' experiences of systematic clinical group supervision and supervised planned nursing care. *Journal of Nursing Management* 8: 357–368.

Bishop, V. 2007. Clinical supervision: What is it? Why do we need it? In Bishop, V. (ed.), *Clinical Supervision in Practice*. 2nd ed. Basingstoke, UK: Palgrave Macmillan, 10–26.

Borton, T. 1970. *Reach, Touch and Teach*. New York: McGraw-Hill.

Brunero, S., Stein-Parbury, J. 2008. The effectiveness of clinical supervision in nursing: An evidence based literature review. *Australian Journal of Advanced Nursing* 25(3): 86–94.

Buus, N., Gonge, H. 2009. Empirical studies of clinical supervision in psychiatric nursing: A systematic literature review and methodological critique. *International Journal of Mental Health Nursing* 18: 250–264.

Care Quality Commission (CQC). 2013. *Supporting Information and Guidance: Supporting Effective Clinical Supervision*. Available from: http://www.cqc.org.uk/sites/default/files/media/documents/20130625_800734_v1_00_supporting_information-effective_clinical_supervision_for_publication.pdf (accessed 24 November 2013).

Chapman, L. 2013. A 'roll-on, roll-off' preceptorship pathway for new registrants. *Nursing Management* 20(2): 24–26.

Courey, T., Benson-Soros, J., Deemer, K., Zeller, R.A. 2006. The missing link: Information literacy and evidence-based practice as a new challenge for nurse educators. *Nursing Education Perspectives* 27(6): 320–323.

Cullum, N., Ciliska, D., Marks, S., Haynes, B. 2008. An introduction to evidence-based nursing. In Cullum, N., Ciliska, D., Marks, S., and Haynes, B. (eds.), *Evidence-Based Nursing: An Introduction*. Oxford, UK: Blackwell, 1–8.

Daylan, A. 2012. Preceptorship: An essential component of qualification. *British Journal of Nursing* 21(10): 613.

Department of Health (DH). 2010. *Preceptorship Framework for Newly Registered Nurses, Midwives and Allied Health Professionals. Nursing.* Gateway reference 13889. Available from: http://webarchive.nationalarchives.gov.uk/20130107105354/http://www.dh.gov.uk/prod_consum_dh/groups/dh_digitalassets/@dh/@en/@abous/documents/digitalasset/dh_114116.pdf (accessed 16 October 2013).

Department of Health (DH). 2013. *The NHS Constitution for England.* Available from: https://www.gov.uk/government/publications/the-nhs-constitution-for-england (accessed 24 November 2013).

Dewey, J. 1929. *Experience and Nature.* New York: Grove Press.

Driscoll, J. 2007. *Practising Clinical Supervision: A Reflective Approach for Healthcare Professionals.* 2nd ed. Edinburgh: Balliere Tindall Elsevier.

Duchscher, J.E. 2009. Transition shock: The initial stage of role adaptation for newly graduated registered nurses. *Journal of Advanced Nursing* 65(5): 1103–1113.

Eason, T. 2010. Lifelong learning: Fostering a culture of curiosity. *Creative Nursing* 16(4): 155–159.

Ford, K., Fitzgerald, M., Courtney-Pratt, H. 2013. The development and evaluation of a preceptorship program using a practice development approach. *Australian Journal of Advanced Nursing* 30(3): 5–13.

Francis, R. 2013. *Report of the Mid Staffordshire NHS Foundation Trust Public Inquiry*. London: Stationery Office.

Gibbs, G. 1988. *Learning by Doing: A Guide to Teaching and Learning Methods.* Further Education Unit. Oxford: Oxford Brookes University.

Gopee, N., 2005. Facilitating the implementation of lifelong learning in nursing. *British Journal of Nursing.* 14(14): 761–767.

Gülmezoglu, A.M, Chandler, J., Shepperd, S., Pantoja, T. 2013. Reviews of qualitative evidence: A new milestone for Cochrane. Available from: http://www.thecochranelibrary.com/details/editorial/5442531/Reviews-of-qualitative-evidence-a-new-milestone-for-Cochrane.html (accessed 10 November 2014).

Harrison-White, K., Simons, J. 2013. Preceptorship: ensuring the best possible start for new nurses. *Nursing Children and Young People* 25(1): 24–27.

Howartson-Jones, L. 2010. *Reflective Practice in Nursing.* Exeter, UK: Learning Matters.

Johns, C. 2013. *Becoming a Reflective Practitioner.* 4th ed. New York: Wiley-Blackwell.

Kolb, D.A. 1984. *Experiential Learning: Experience as the Source of Learning and Development.* London: Prentice Hall International.

Kolb, D.A., Fry, R. 1975. Towards an applied theory of experiential learning. In Cooper, C.L. (ed.), *Theories of Group Processes.* London: Wiley, 33–57.

Langley, G.J., Moen, R.D., Nolan, K.M., et al. 2009. *The Improvement Guide: A Practical Approach to Enhancing Organizational Performance.* 2nd ed. San Francisco: Jossey-Bass.

Lawler, J. 1991. *Behind the Screens: Nursing Somology and the Problem of the Body.* London: Churchill Livingstone.

Leigh, J.A., Douglas, C.H., Lee, K., Douglas, M.R. 2005. A case study of a preceptorship programme in an acute NHS trust–using the European Foundation for Quality Management tool to support clinical practice development. *Journal of Nursing Management* 13: 508–518.

Morgan, A., Mattison, J., Stephens, M. 2012. Implementing structured preceptorship in an acute hospital. *Nursing Standard* 26(28): 35–39.

NHS Institute for Innovation and Improvement. 2009. *Your Skin Matters.* Available from: http://www.institute.nhs.uk/building_capability/hia_supporting_info/your_skin_matters.html (accessed 10 November 2013).

NHS Staff Council. 2013. *NHS Terms and Conditions of Service Handbook Amendment Number 29 Pay Circular (AforC) 3/2013.* Available from: http://www.nhsemployers.org/SiteCollectionDocuments/afc_tc_of_service_handbook_fb.pdf (accessed 16 October 2013).

Norris, N. 2010. How to ... carry out a literature search. *Education for Primary Care* 21: 124–25.

Nursing and Midwifery Council (NMC). 2008. *The Code: Standards for Conduct, Performance and Ethics for Nurses and Midwives.* London: NMC.

Nursing and Midwifery Council (NMC). 2011. *The Prep Handbook.* Available from: http://www.nmc-uk.org/Documents/Standards/NMC_Prep-handbook_2011.pdf (accessed 16 October 2013).

Nursing and Midwifery Council (NMC). 2013. *Revalidation.* Available from: http://www.nmc-uk.org/Nurses-and-midwives/Revalidation/ (accessed 24 November 2013).

Palmer, A., Burns, S., Bulam, C. 1994. *Reflective Practice in Nursing: The Growth of the Reflective Practitioner.* Oxford, UK: Blackwell Science.

Petaloti, S. 2009. Lifelong learning in nursing science and practice: A bibliographic review. *Hellenic Journal of Nursing Science* 2(2): 45–47.

Proctor, B. 1986. Supervision: A co-operative exercise in accountability. In Marken, M., and Payne, M. (eds.), *Enabling and Ensuring: Supervision in Practice.* Leicester, UK: Leicester National Youth Bureau and Council for Education and Training in Youth and Community Work, 21–23.

Royal College of Nursing (RCN). 2005. *NHS Knowledge and Skills Framework Outlines for Nursing Posts.* London: RCN.

Schön, D. 1991. *The Reflective Practitioner.* Aldershot, UK: Ashgate.

Schön, D. 1987. *Educating the Reflective Practitioner.* San Francisco: Jossey-Bass.

Wigens, L., Heathershaw, R. 2013. *Mentorship and Clinical Supervision Skills in Health Care.* Andover, MA: Cengage Learning.

Index

Note: Page numbers ending in "f" refer to figures. Page numbers ending in "t" refer to tables.

Index

D

E

Index

Index

Index

O

P

Index